The management of genital warts in primary care

Margaret Stanley
Jane Sterling
Chris Sonnex

British Library Cataloguing in Publication Data. A catalogue record for
this title is available from the British Library

ISBN 1-904218-07-5

Design and production:
Design Online Limited, 21 Cave Street, Oxford OX4 1BA, UK

Printed by
Ingoprint, Barcelona, Spain

Distributed by
Plymbridge Distributors Ltd, Estover Road, Plymouth PL6 7PY, UK

The management of genital warts in primary care

Contents

Chapter 1

Genital warts: an overview

Chris Sonnex

Historical context

There have been writings since the first century AD describing the clinical features of what we now recognize as genital warts. The Greek physician Galen wrote that 'The "thymus" is a rough looking elevation, which all alike show themselves upon the genitals and about the anus'. The term 'thymus', meaning mulberry-like, was used for describing any ano-genital lump and Rufus of Ephesus (AD 90–11) attempted to differentiate between 'broad' and 'pointed' thymi. The term 'ficus', meaning a fig, also appeared in the early Greek literature and descriptions of patients with 'fig warts' continued in many European countries up to the nineteenth and early twentieth centuries. The term 'condyloma', meaning 'a round swelling adjacent to the anus' was introduced by the ancient Greeks, with the more familiar term 'condyloma acuminatum' or 'pointed condyloma' appearing only towards the end of the nineteenth century. Fallopius made the distinction between condylomata acuminata and condylomata lata (a feature of secondary syphilis) in the mid-sixteenth century.

Epidemiology

Genital warts are the commonest sexually transmitted infection diagnosed in the developing world. During 2000 there were 570 000 new diagnoses made in genitourinary (GU) medicine clinics in the UK (see Figure 1.1). Twenty per cent (112 000) were patients with a first episode or recurrences of

Figure 1.1.
Rates (per 100 000 population) of diagnoses of genital warts (first episode) made in GU medicine clinics by sex and country for the UK (1995–2000).

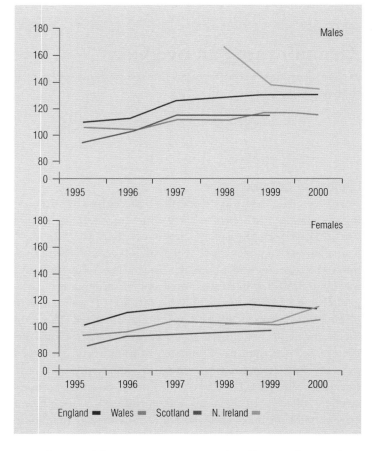

genital warts. This represents a rise of 17% over the previous 5 years. The highest rates are found in the 20–24 and 16–24 year age groups for males and females, respectively. The overall rates are distributed uniformly across the UK for both males and females.

The epidemiology of genital warts represents the epidemiology of clinical disease caused by human papillomavirus (HPV) types 6 and 11 (for information on viral types, see page 81). Data from the UK and Scandinavia have shown incidence rates of 0.5–2% in young men and women aged 18–25 years of age.

Considering ano-genital HPV infection in general (i.e. clinical and subclinical infection), the incidence rates have been reported as being 47.1 and 50.5 infections per 100 person years in females and males, respectively. Incidence rates of cervico-vaginal infection of 10–20% have been reported in women in their early twenties. The prevalence of cervical infection decreases after 30 years of age. There is inevitably some variation between studies owing to differences in the age and demographic characteristics of the populations studied and the methods of HPV identification used.

The disease spectrum of ano-genital human papillomavirus infection

A wide disease spectrum of ano-genital HPV infection is now recognized. Genital warts and some dysplastic lesions are clinically apparent, although small lesions may only be appreciated by using some form of magnification such as the colposcope. Subclinical disease is considered 100 times more common than clinically overt disease and may be detected by the following means.

Application of acetic acid

HPV-infected epithelium often whitens following the application of an acetic acid solution. This is called 'aceto-whitening' and is most commonly used for identifying cervical disease, in particular dysplastic lesions (cervical intra-epithelial neoplasia or CIN), although the method may be applied to any ano-genital site. A 3–5% acetic acid solution is used, usually by means of a gauze swab or cotton wool ball soaked in the solution. The time taken for the epithelium to whiten varies from 20 to 60 s for the cervix and anal canal to approximately 3–5 min for the vulva, penis and peri-anal skin. Although suggestive of HPV infection, aceto-whitening is not specific and may be seen with inflammatory conditions. Magnified examination of aceto-white lesions may reveal characteristic features such as capillary punctation. However, biopsy and histological examination are usually required in order to make a definitive diagnosis (see Figure 1.2).

Keypoints

* incidence rates are 0.5–2% in the 18–25 years age group

* incidence rate of ano-genital HPV infection are reported as being 47.1 and 50.5 infections per 100 person years in males and females respectively

Figure 1.2.
(a) Cervical aceto-whitening: HPV infection found on biopsy and histology (see Figure 1.3).
(b) Cervical aceto-whitening: CIN grade 3 on histology.
(c) Vulval aceto-whitening: non-specific.
(d) Vulval wart: appearance accentuated by aceto-whitening.

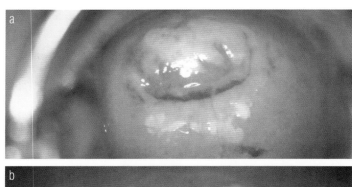

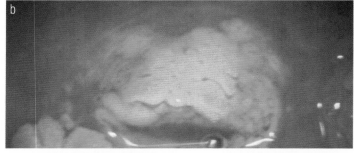

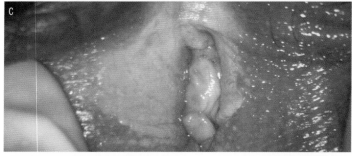

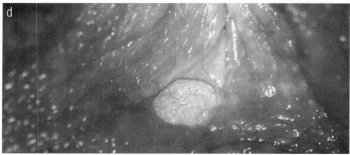

Cytology and histology

HPV-infected cells and tissue display certain characteristic features. Koilocytosis is considered the diagnostic hallmark of HPV infection. A koilocyte is a squamous epithelial cell showing enlargement and rounding of the cell outline together with peripheral condensation of the cytoplasm leading to a clear space or halo around the nucleus. The nucleus is also usually hyperchromatic or may be enlarged with a fine, pale chromatin pattern. The nuclear outline is often crenated and cells may be binucleate or multinucleate (Figure 1.3).

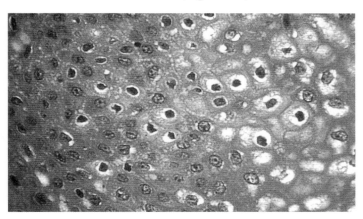

Figure 1.3
HPV-infected epithelium showing koilocytes.

Human papillomavirus DNA detection

An HPV-infected epithelium may fail to whiten with acetic acid and have a normal cytological/histological appearance. However, HPV DNA may still be detected by means of molecular techniques such as *in situ* hybridization or the polymerase chain reaction (PCR). The PCR enables small amounts of DNA to be amplified enormously making subsequent characterization possible. This method has been used in many epidemiological studies of HPV infection.

Keypoint

✳ 'Aceto-whitening' is most commonly used method for identifying cervical disease, in particular dysplastic lesions

Natural history

HPV infects the basal layer of the genital epithelium. Its replication is closely linked to the maturation of the keratinocyte, with infectious virus appearing only in the most differentiated superficial cells of the epithelium. Transcription of HPV genes in the nude mouse model takes place approximately 4 weeks after initial infection, with warts appearing after 10–12 weeks. The incubation period for genital warts is 3 weeks to 8 months, with the majority of lesions developing at 2–3 months. Once warts have developed they may show minimal change over time, become more numerous or larger or regress spontaneously. Although most studies have suggested minimal regression in the short term, some have recorded up to 30% regression within 3 months.[1] The rate of long-term spontaneous regression is not known. Recurrence is common following wart clearance with rates of between 25 and 67% within 3 months. HPV may persist in the epithelium in the absence of clinically apparent warts and, while this latent infection may persist throughout life, there is some evidence to suggest that it may be cleared with time. Many patients ask whether they can transmit the virus when warts are not present. The answer is probably yes, but the degree of infectivity of subclinical HPV infection is unknown.

Diagnosis

Genital warts are usually diagnosed by their clinical appearance. Biopsy is reserved for atypical lesions, particularly if intra-epithelial neoplasia is suspected. Ano-genital HPV infection is multifocal with lesions more commonly appearing at sites of 'trauma' or greatest friction during sexual intercourse. Although solitary warts are sometimes seen, lesions are usually multiple and may coalesce to form large plaques. Extensive warts are particularly seen in immunosuppressed patients and usually prove difficult to clear.

Warts in men

Penis

The most commonly affected sites in uncircumcised men are the glans penis, inner aspect of the foreskin, coronal sulcus and frenulum. The penile shaft is more frequently affected in circumcised men. Urethral and/or meatal warts have been found in between 5 and 23% of men with penile warts. Warts beyond the terminal 1 cm of the urethra are uncommon and bladder condylomata are very rare. Urethral and meatal warts are often asymptomatic, although occasionally patients may present with bleeding or dysuria. Meatoscopy is a useful method for detecting intra-meatal and distal urethral warts. An auroscope may be used for this purpose, although in the clinical setting a better view is obtained by using a colposcope and aural speculum. If there is clinical suspicion urethral ultrasound, urethroscopy or urethrography may be used for detecting more proximal urethral lesions (see Figure 1.4).

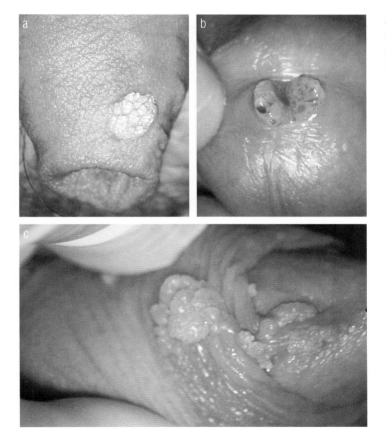

Figure 1.4
(a) Penile wart.
(b) Meatal wart.
(c) Preputal warts.

Anus

Anal warts have been reported to be several times more common than penile warts in homosexual men, with lesions often extending into the anal canal. Although anal intercourse increases the risk of acquiring anal HPV infection it is by no means a prerequisite. Anal warts are well recognized in heterosexual men and have been reported in 30–45% of those with penile warts. In one study one-third of men were unaware of their presence. The method of viral transmission to the anus in heterosexual men is uncertain and, although one study looked at the possibility of finger transmission, this was not confirmed. Warts beyond the squamo-columnar junction or dentate line are rare. The precursor of anal squamous cell carcinoma, anal intra-epithelial neoplasia grade 3 (AIN III), is associated predominantly with HPV type 16 infection and originates at the squamo-columnar junction, a feature in common with CIN. Colposcopic examination of the anal canal via a proctoscope is an excellent way of detecting both warts and AIN lesions (see Figure 1.5). Human immunodeficiency virus (HIV)-infected homosexual men are at particular risk of developing AIN III.

Warts in women

Genital warts in women are most commonly found in the vestibulum, on the labia and at the posterior fourchette of the vulva. The urethral meatus is affected in 4–8% of females, less commonly than in men. Cervical warts have been documented in 6–8% of women with genital warts, vaginal warts in 10–15% and anal warts in approximately 20%. Most cervical HPV infection is subclinical and may be detected by cervical cytology or colposcopic examination following the application of acetic acid (see Figure 1.6).

Wart types

Warts on mucosal surfaces and under the prepuce are usually pink–red and non-keratinized. Warts on the penile shaft and hair-bearing skin are usually grey or brown and keratinized. Warts tend to be non-pigmented, but, if so, are mostly seen on the labia

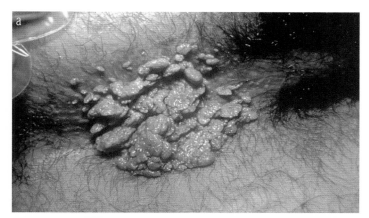

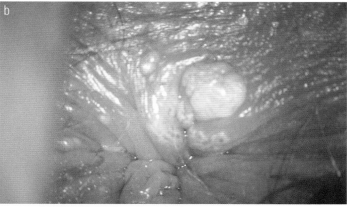

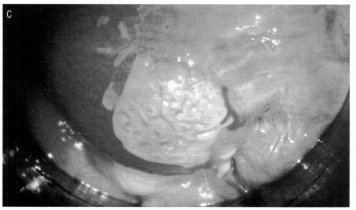

*Figure 1.5
(a) Peri-anal warts.
(b) Peri-anal warts.
(c) Anal canal
warts (post-
application of
acetic acid).*

Figure 1.6
(a) Vulval warts.
(b) Vulval warts.
(c) Introital warts.
(d) Cervical warts.
(e) Cervical warts
and CIN.

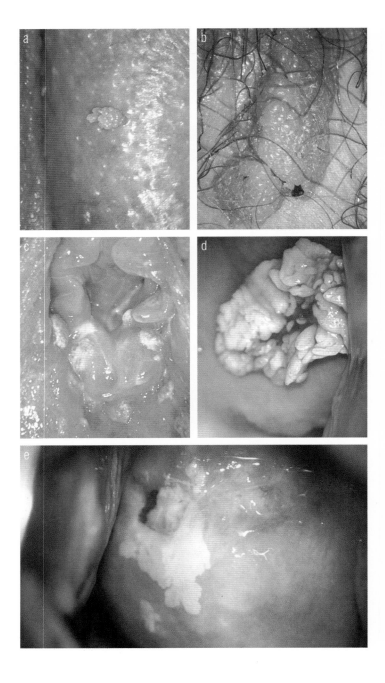

majora, penile shaft, pubis, groin, perineum and peri-anal area. Whether warts are keratinized or non-keratinized may determine which is the most appropriate method of treatment.

There are three major types of wart morphology.

Condylomata acuminata

This term is used for describing warts that have a pointed, irregular, fissured appearance – the so-called 'classical wart'. They are highly vascular and show an obvious punctated or capillary pattern on mucosal surfaces. They may coalesce to form large plaques or cauliflower-like lesions, an appearance seen particularly in pregnancy and in immunosuppressed patients, such as those with HIV infection or following organ transplantation (see Figure 1.7).

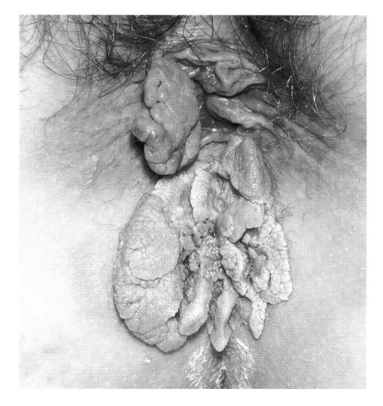

Figure 1.7
Extensive vulval warts in a patient post-renal transplantation.

Papular warts

These are most common on keratinized epithelium and are often hyperkeratotic with a smooth surface. They may be multiple and usually stay as separate lesions. Pigmented papular lesions should be biopsied in order to exclude penile or vulval intra-epithelial neoplasia (PIN or VIN) (see Figure 1.8).

Figure 1.8
Papular warts
affecting the penile
shaft.

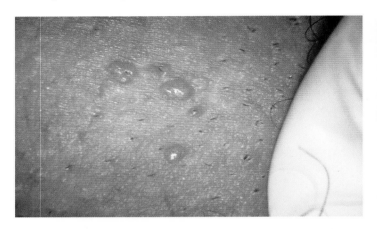

Macular or flat lesions

These are usually found on mucosal surfaces and may be difficult to identify with the naked eye because of only subtle colour variation. The application of acetic acid and colposcopic examination may be required for identifying the slightly raised edge and the characteristic presence of capillary punctation (see Figure 1.9). Biopsy is often needed for confirming the diagnosis and for excluding PIN or VIN.

Buschke–Löwenstein tumour and verrucous carcinoma

The giant condylomas, which were first described by Buschke and Löwenstein in 1925, are very uncommon. They are caused by HPV types 6 and 11 and usually present as single, large, foul-smelling, cauliflower-like masses. They are typically slow growing and are prone to recurrences. Histologically they show both a downward and upward growth pattern and in the anal region may penetrate into the peri-rectal tissue and

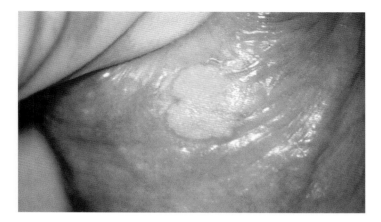

*Figure 1.9
Macular HPV
lesion affecting the
penis: appearance
accentuated by
the application of
acetic acid.*

rectal wall. Dysplastic change may occur and so long-term follow-up post-treatment is advised.

Verrucous carcinoma is considered a low-grade and well-differentiated variant of squamous cell carcinoma. Although lesions tend to remain localized and follow an indolent course, metastases may occur. There is still some uncertainty whether Buschke–Löwenstein tumours and verrucous carcinomas are truly separate entities.

Differential diagnosis of genital warts

The commonest causes of misdiagnosis are hirsuties papillaris penis in men, vulval micropapillae in women and Fordyce spots and molluscum contagiosum in both sexes.

Hirsuties papillaris penis (pearly penile papules)

These are small dome-shaped or conical-shaped lesions present around the corona of the glans penis (see Figure 1.10). They usually appear during adolescence and have been reported in up to almost 50% of men. In most men the papules are less than 1 mm in diameter and may be hardly noticeable. However, occasionally they can be larger and quite extensive which may cause concern and embarrassment. Although no treatment is generally recommended, men with marked psychological problems may benefit from cryotherapy or laser ablation of the papules.

Figure 1.10
Hirsuties papillaris
penis (pearly penile
papules).

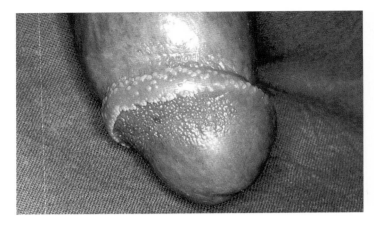

Vulval micropapillae

Small finger-like projections or papillae are present on the inner surface of the labia minora in a large proportion of women (see Figure 1.11). They are anatomical variants of the normal vulvar epithelium and vary appreciably in size and number. Careful examination with magnification, such as a colposcope, may be required for accurate identification. Some years ago HPV was thought to play a possible causative role. However, this has not been substantiated by more recent studies.

Figure 1.11
Vulval micropapillae.

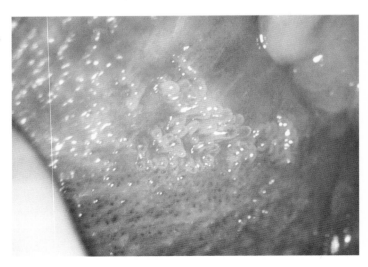

Fordyce spots

These are sebaceous glands present on the inner surface of the prepuce and labia minora. They are common and appear as small, smooth, multiple, discrete greyish-yellow lesions (see Figure 1.12).

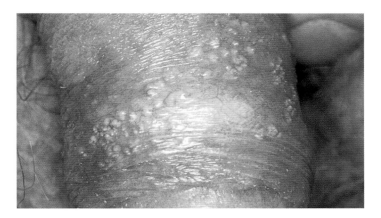

Figure 1.12
Fordyce spots.

Molluscum contagiosum

Caused by a member of the poxvirus family (molluscum contagiosum virus), this presents as small rounded papules, characteristically with a small central punctum (see Figure 1.13). This central pit may be more easily seen on spraying the lesion with liquid nitrogen, which is the recommended method of treatment.

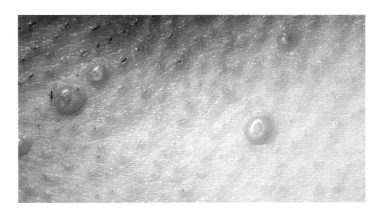

Figure 1.13
Molluscum
contagiosum.

Fibroepitheliomata

Skin tags of a variety of sizes affect the ano-genital skin (see Figure 1.14). Removal by scissor excision is recommended only if there is diagnostic uncertainty or if lesions catch on underwear or look unsightly to the individual.

Figure 1.14
Vulval skin tag.

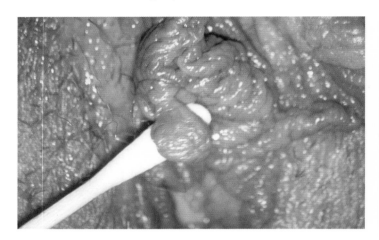

Seborrhoeic keratoses

These are occasionally found on the genital skin and may be difficult to distinguish from keratinized papular warts (see Figure 1.15).

Figure 1.15
Penile seborrhoeic
keratoses.

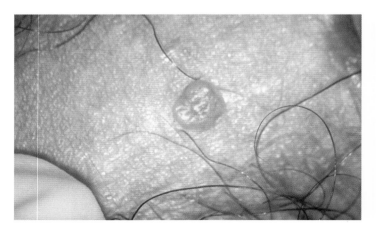

Lichen planus

Small papular lesions of lichen planus may closely resemble papular warts (see Figure 1.16). Biopsy may be required in order to distinguish between the two accurately.

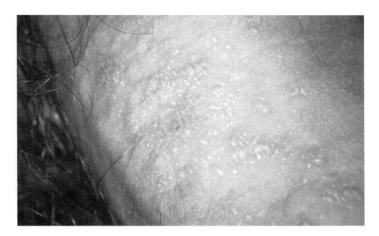

*Figure 1.16
Penile lichen
planus.*

Condylomata lata

These are a feature of secondary syphilis and present as raised pink or grey papular lesions usually affecting warm, moist areas, such as the perineum and peri-anal skin (see Figure 1.17). Syphilis serology would be strongly positive at the time when condylomata lata start to develop.

Key points

1. Genital warts are the commonest sexually transmitted infection diagnosed in the developing world.
2. The highest rates are found in the 20–24 and 16–24 year age groups for males and females, respectively.
3. Subclinical HPV infection is considered 100 times more common than clinically overt disease.
4. The incubation period for genital warts is 3 weeks to 8 months, with the majority of lesions developing at 2–3 months. Incubation periods of greater than one year have been anecdotally reported.

Figure 1.17
Peri-anal
condylomata lata.

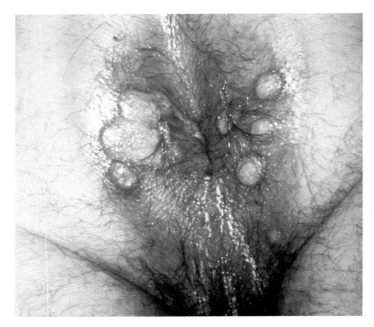

5. The majority of genital warts are acquired as a result of sexual intercourse. Hand wart HPV types have been reported to cause genital lesions in children, but this is uncommon in adults.
6. Genital warts are usually diagnosed by clinical appearance. Biopsy is reserved for atypical lesions, particularly if intra-epithelial neoplasia is suspected.
7. Anal warts are well recognized in heterosexual men and have been reported in 30–45% of those with penile warts.

Reference

1. Ho GYF, Bierman R, Beardsley L *et al.* Natural history of cervicovaginal papillomavirus infection in young women. *N Engl J Med* 1998; **338**: 423–8.

Chapter 2
Biology of the papillomaviruses

Margaret Stanley

Introduction and history

The humble wart has a long and honourable history, with clinical descriptions of these excrescences as long ago as Greek and Roman times. The Italian physician Ciuffo showed the infectious nature of warts unequivocally in 1907 by demonstrating person-to-person transmission of lesions by cell-free, wart filtrates – a study unlikely to meet with ethical approval today. Richard Shope identified the first animal papillomavirus, the cottontail rabbit virus (CRPV), which caused skin warts or papillomas on rabbits, in the 1930s. This was seminal work, establishing key aspects of papillomavirus pathogenesis, including the oncogenic potential of this group of viruses.

As the electron microscope began to be used as a research tool in biology in the 1950s, papillomaviruses were revealed to be the infectious agent for human warts. However, although papillomaviruses were shown to have a genome consisting of circular double-stranded DNA in 1964, biochemical characterization of their proteins was slow because there was no tissue culture system for virus growth available. Virus particles had to be obtained from clinical lesions and, to inhibit matters further, the amount of virus in warts was highly variable. For example, virions were abundant in plantar warts, but sparse in laryngeal and genital warts. These handicaps severely limited immunological and virological studies and, until the mid-1970s, the general view was that there was only one human papillomavirus (HPV) and that tissue location rather than virus type dictated the morphology and behaviour of the clinical lesions at a specific epithelial surface.

The advent of recombinant DNA technology and molecular cloning completely reversed this view, revealing what is an astonishing plurality of both human and animal papillomaviruses. Papillomaviruses it turned out were exquisitely tissue trophic and the different clinical lesions were in fact distinct diseases caused by infection with specific groups of HPV types (Table 2.1). In addition, the viruses were shown to be absolutely species specific, such that HPVs could only infect humans, rabbit papillomaviruses only rabbits and so on. It became clear that, within a species, the individual viruses showed a predilection for either skin or internal squamous mucosae and that, within the groups of skin or mucosal viruses, they could be separated into high- or low-risk types depending upon their oncogenic potential. The genital tract illustrated this dramatically. Genital warts were shown to be predominantly associated with HPV 6 and 11, viruses that were almost never detected in carcinomas, whereas HPV 16 and 18 and their close relatives were associated with intra-epithelial lesions, particularly in the cervix and were detected in more than 90% of cervix cancers.[1]

Viral genome organization and virus structure

Papillomaviruses are minnows in the virus world and the virus particle or virion consists of a protein coat encapsidating a circular DNA molecule of approximately 8000 base pairs (8 kb) in size, which is tiny compared to pox or herpes viruses. The genome can be divided into three domains. The first is a short stretch of DNA (the length differs between different HPV types) known by various names: the non-coding region, the long control region or the upstream regulatory region. As these names indicate this region does not encode any genes, but controls the expression of the eight viral genes that make up the remainder of the genome. In order to do this the non-coding region contains short DNA sequences or motifs that bind both cellular and viral proteins known as transcription

Keypoints

* until the mid-1970s, the general view was that there was only one human papillomavirus

* DNA technology and molecular cloning revealed an astonishing plurality of both human and animal papillomaviruses

Lesion	HPV types	
	Frequent association	Infrequent association
Skin warts		
Plantar warts	1	2, 4 & 63
Common warts	2 & 27	1, 4, 7, 26, 28, 29, 57, 60, 65
Flat warts	3 & 10	2, 26, 27, 28, 29, 41, 49
Epidermodysplasia verruci-formis-specific skin lesions	5, 8, 17 & 20	9, 12, 14, 15, 19, 21-25, 36,38, 46, 47 & 50
Malignant and pre-malignant skin lesions		
Bowen's disease of the skin	2, 16 & 34	–
Skin cancers in patients with epidermodysplasia verruciformis	5 & 8	14, 17, 20 & 47
Skin cancers in renal transplant patients	1–6, 8, 10, 11, 14–16, 18–20, 23–25, 27, 29, 36, 38, 41, 47 & 48	–
Squamous cell carcinoma of the finger	16	–
Benign head and neck lesions		
Oral papillomas and leukoplakias	2, 6, 11 & 16	7
Focal epithelial hyperplasia	13 & 32	–
Laryngeal papillomas (RRP patients)	6 & 11	–
Conjunctival papillomas	6 & 11	–
Nasal papillomas	–	6, 11 & 57
Malignant head and neck lesions		
Laryngeal cancer	–	6, 11, 16, 18 & 35
Oral cancer	–	3, 6, 11, 16, 18 & 57
Tonsillar/Pharyngeal cancer	–	16, 18 & 33
Oesophageal cancer	–	6, 11, 16 & 18
Nasal cancer	–	16 & 57
Benign ano-genital lesions		
Condyloma acuminata	6 & 11	30, 34, 33, 40, 41, 42, 44, 42, 44, 45, 54, 55 & 61
Malignant and pre-malignant ano-genital lesions		
CIN, PAIN, PIN, VAIN and VIN	6, 11, 16, 18 & 31	30, 34, 35, 39, 40, 42–45, 51, 52, 56–59, 61, 62, 64, 66, 67, & 69
Cervical cancer	16, 18, 31 & 45	6, 10, 11, 26, 33, 35, 39, 51, 52, 55, 56, 58, 59, 66 & 68, plus unclassified types
Non-cervical ano-genital cancers	6, 16 & 18	11, 31 & 33

CIN, cervical intra-epithelial neoplasia; PAIN, peri-anal intra-epithelial neoplasia; PIN, penile intra-epithelial neoplasia; RRP, recurrent respiratory papillomatosis; VAIN, vaginal intra-epithelial neoplasia; VIN, vulval intra-epithelial neoplasia.

Table 2.1.
Clinical lesions associated with HPV

factors: this binding can either turn on or turn off gene expression by activating or repressing the promoter of the gene. Transcription factors do not function individually but in combination and the combinatorial composition of the complex is therefore the key determinant as to whether a particular gene is expressed or not. Since papillomaviruses are regulated by cellular as well as viral transcription factors this permits a sophisticated level of control, reflecting the state of cellular differentiation. This control is further refined by the fact that different viral promoters are activated at different stages of the life cycle with both early and late promoters. The second region of the genome encodes the early genes E1, E2 and E4–E7, which express proteins essential for viral replication. The third region, the late region, encodes the viral capsid proteins L1 and L2. A genomic map of HPV 6 is shown in Figure 2.1 and a brief description of the functions of the different viral proteins is given in Table 2.2.

Figure 2.1.
A circular map of the genome of HPV 6. The early genes encode functions that are important for the establishment of infection and the initiation of viral replication. The late genes encode the coat or capsid proteins of the virus. The long control region contains transcriptional control elements and the origin of viral DNA replication. Although the viruses are composed of double-stranded DNA transcription occurs from only one strand in one direction.

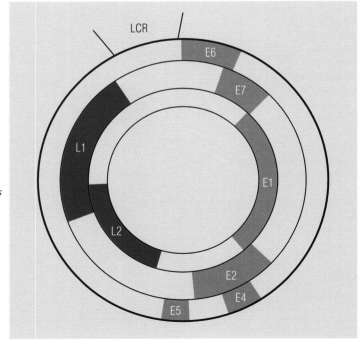

Gene	Function
E6	High-risk HPV E6 binds p53 and directs p53 ubiquitin-mediated degradation With high-risk HPV E7 immortalizes primary keratinocytes
E7	High-risk HPV E7 binds pRb and deregulates the G_1/S cell cycle checkpoint Cooperates with E6 in immortalizing primary cells
E1	The only viral enzyme: a helicase and ATPase and an ATP-binding protein essential for viral DNA replication
E2	The viral transcription factor: binds E1 in order to facilitate the initiation of viral DNA replication and is also important in genome encapsidation
E5	Up-regulates growth factor receptors and is possibly involved in immune evasion by down-regulating major histocompatibility complex protein expression
E4	Interacts with cytoskeletal proteins, allows viral assembly and inhibits cellular DNA but not viral DNA replication
L1	Major capsid protein
L2	Minor capsid protein

Table 2.2
The functions of
HPV genes

High-resolution electron microscopy reveals the virion to be a particle of approximately 55 nm in diameter (Figure 2.2). The protein coat, which encloses the DNA genome, is assembled from 72 individual units or capsomers. These are pentamers and are composed predominantly of the L1 protein with L2 embedded deep within the protein shell. It is thought that L1 contains the ligand for the cellular receptor for the virus and that the major neutralizing epitope against which serum-neutralizing antibodies are generated is within L1.

Classification of human papillomaviruses

Papillomaviruses are classified by genotype, i.e. DNA sequence, not by serotype and a new HPV type is recognized if the L1 region of the DNA sequences cloned from a clinical lesion differs by more than 10% from a known HPV. At the present time more than 130 such HPVs have been described but, although there are a plethora of HPV types, fortunately only a small number are found commonly in clinical lesions in the genital tract (Table 2.1). Having said this, mixed infections are common in the genital tract, particularly in intra-epithelial

Figure 2.2
A high-resolution
electron
micrograph of
negatively stained
papillomavirus
particles.
The virion is
approximately
55 nm in diameter.

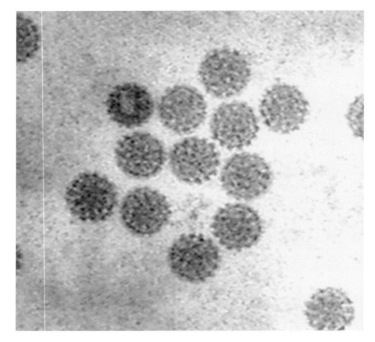

lesions, but again a single type usually dominates and, although the DNA of more than one type may be detected, viral transcripts and viral proteins generally come from only one type within the lesion. The phylogenetic relationships between HPV types based on genome sequence variation indicate how these viruses have evolved and their relationship to each other. Interestingly, the clinical distinctions between skin and mucosal warts and benign and malignant lesions correlate with the virus phylogenetic tree, as modelled by computer (Figure 2.3).

The infectious cycle

The virus life cycle is the key to understanding the pathogenesis of papillomavirus-associated disease. These viruses have an absolutely restricted host range and tissue specificity and, in the natural infection, HPVs only infect human keratinocytes or cells with the potential for squamous maturation such as

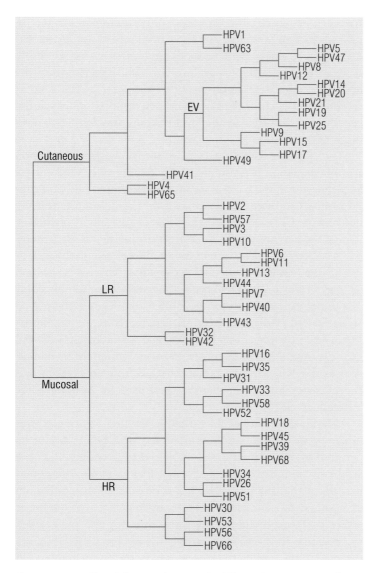

Figure 2.3
A phylogenetic tree
of 48 HPV types
based on the E6
gene sequences
constructed by
Van Ranst et
al.2 The viruses
cluster together
into cutaneous and
mucosal groups
and fall into
high- and low-risk
types within these
groups.

the reserve cells of the uterine cervix. There is no tissue culture
system that supports a complete infectious cycle, i.e. infection
of cells in culture with virus and the subsequent generation
and release of new infectious virus particles. What is the basis

for such tropism? Interestingly, cultured human or mouse fibroblasts will take up virus or virus-like particles (geometrically correct empty protein shells generated by self-assembly of L1 protein or L1 plus L2 protein). This suggests that the host and tissue restriction is not at the level of the cellular receptor, but is controlled by the transcriptional milieu of the cell and possibly also at the level of translation of RNA messages into proteins.

The complete infectious cycle is absolutely dependent upon the differentiation programme of the keratinocyte. Virus infects keratinocytes in the basal layer of the epithelium, but viral capsid proteins and virus particles are only assembled in terminally differentiated keratinocytes. The virus is basically a hitchhiker joining the keratinocyte at the start of its journey from a primitive basal cell (probably a stem cell) in the epithelium through to its end as a terminally differentiated squame. This is a replication strategy in which viral DNA replication and virus assembly occur in a cell already destined for death by natural causes: there is no virus-induced cytolysis or necrosis and, therefore, no inflammation. Our knowledge of the temporal and spatial patterns of viral gene expression comes mainly from natural infections in animals such as the dog, cow and rabbit, but also from an experimental rodent xenograft system that was first used for examining the infectious cycle of HPV 11.[3]

Overall these studies show that, in the first 3–4 weeks after infection with large amounts of virus, viral DNA cannot be detected by *in situ* hybridization.[4] This suggests that either the viral copy number in infected cells is below five to ten copies per cell or that the infected cell is a rare cell in the epithelium or both! At 4–5 weeks viral DNA can be detected in the lower layers of the epithelium and transcripts for the early genes are present. At 5–8 weeks strong signals for viral DNA are detected in the middle to upper layers of the epithelium and in some cells the viral copy number can be in the order of 1000 copies or more per cell. E6 and E7 mRNAs are present at low levels in the lower dividing epithelial layers, but are highly abundant in the upper differentiating layers. At approximately

8 weeks post-infection L1 and L2 capsid protein expression can be detected in the most superficial cells of the epithelium. The sequence of events for one of these experimental models, the canine oral papillomavirus (COPV), a low-risk mucosal virus infecting the oropharynx of dogs,[5] is shown in Figure 2.4. A similar spatial and temporal pattern of gene expression is observed in HPV 6- or 11-infected genital warts, but expression of the early genes E6 and E7 is less abundant in the basal and parabasal cells and viral DNA can only be detected by *in situ* hybridization in suprabasal cells[4] (Figure 2.5). However, in lesions caused by HPV 16 and the other high-risk HPVs early gene expression is under very tight control: E6 and E7 transcripts are barely detectable in the basal and parabasal layers and are expressed abundantly only in the upper stratum spinosum and granulosum.

The best scenario for the infectious cycle (Figure 2.6) seems to be the following. Virus infects a subset of primitive basal epithelial cells, probably stem cells, at a low copy number. At some time after infection there is a round of viral DNA replication amplifying the viral copy number to approximately 50 copies per cell. It is speculated that this initial round of viral DNA replication is independent of the cell cycle and may occur in a cell out of cycle. The infected keratinocyte probably then leaves the stem cell compartment moving first laterally in the basal layer and then upwards into the lower spinous layers. These cells are actively dividing and here the virus maintains a constant copy number replicating the episome when the cell divides. This phase of the life cycle is described as plasmid or episomal maintenance and, during this period, viral gene expression, particularly for the high-risk viruses, is minimal. Next the infected keratinocyte enters the differentiating compartment of the epithelium exiting the cell cycle. This coincides with a massive up-regulation of viral gene expression and viral DNA replication. There is amplification of the viral copy number to at least 1000 copies per cell, abundant expression of all the early genes and expression of the late genes L1 and L2.

*Figure 2.4
Gene expression in
the COPV infectious
cycle. Viral DNA
cannot be detected by
in situ hybridization
until 3–4 weeks after
infection with the
virus. Viral DNA is
first detected at week 4
in tight clusters of cells
each arising from a
rete ridge. At 6 weeks
almost all basal and
most suprabasal cells
are viral DNA positive
with the strongest
signals in sporadic cells
in the superficial layers
with the morphology
of koilocytes. At week
9, when the wart is
regressing, viral DNA
is lost from the basal
layers, but is retained
in the tips of the wart
papillae. Transcripts
for the E7 gene
parallel viral DNA
expression in weeks
5–7, but expression
is not strong in the
superficial layers
where only sporadic
cells exhibit strong
signals. The L1 and
L2 genes are not
expressed until weeks
7–8 and transcripts
are confined to
superficial cells with
the morphology of the
koilocytes.[5]*

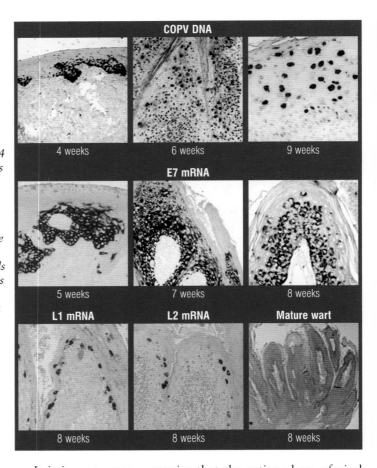

It is important to recognize that the active phase of viral DNA replication and amplification of viral copy number is occurring in cells that are differentiating and have exited the cell cycle. The papillomaviruses encode only one enzyme, namely E1, a DNA helicase and, apart from this and the E2 protein that cooperates with E1 in binding to the viral origin of replication, viral DNA synthesis is totally dependent upon the cellular DNA synthetic machinery. The problem for the virus is that the cellular proteins involved in DNA synthesis, the polymerases and accessory proteins, are expressed only in

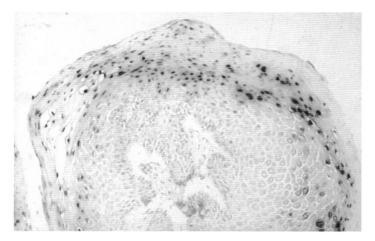

Figure 2.5 DNA:DNA in situ hybridization of an HPV 6-containing genital wart. In contrast to the COPV wart, viral DNA can be detected only in the suprabasal and superficial layers of the infected epithelium.

mitotically active cells. In order to solve this the virus encodes proteins that, in the context of the viral life cycle, reactivate cellular DNA synthesis in non-cycling cells and delay the differentiation programme of the infected keratinocyte, thereby creating an environment permissive for viral DNA replication. The precise details by which this is achieved are imperfectly understood, but the viral genes central to these functions are E6 and E7. An unfortunate but rare by-product of this role in the life cycle of the E6 and E7 genes of the oncogenic HPVs is the inappropriate expression of these genes in dividing cells and the development of cancer.[6]

Target cell for infection

The dependence upon the keratinocyte lineage for viral gene expression extends to the target cell for infection. In experimental CRPV infections, viral gene transcription is detected first in the hair follicle, in cells that have the characteristics of stem cells.[7] This is also true in COPV where viral DNA amplification and early gene transcription are first detected at the extreme tips of the rete ridges (Figure 2.4), which are thought to be the site of interfollicular keratinocyte stem cells.[5] If the target cell for infection is the stem cell then this does offer an explanation for some interesting aspects of papillomavirus

Figure 2.6
The infectious cycle
of HPV.

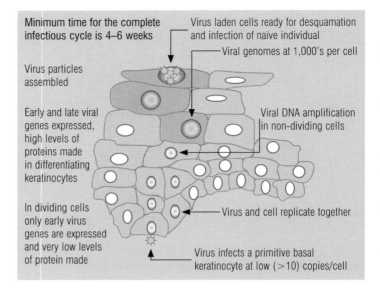

Minimum time for the complete infectious cycle is 4–6 weeks

Virus laden cells ready for desquamation and infection of naïve individual

Viral genomes at 1,000's per cell

Virus particles assembled

Early and late viral genes expressed, high levels of proteins made in differentiating keratinocytes

Viral DNA amplification in non-dividing cells

In dividing cells only early virus genes are expressed and very low levels of protein made

Virus and cell replicate together

Virus infects a primitive basal keratinocyte at low (>10) copies/cell

biology. There is for example the phenomenon of the lag phase between infection and the first detection of viral DNA and early gene expression. The length of this lag in experimental models such as the rabbit, the dog and rodent xenografts of HPV 11 and HPV 16 is consistently between 3 and 5 weeks. Anecdotal evidence in man suggests a similar time lag for genital warts.[8] One could speculate that the virus infects a resting stem cell held in the G_0 phase of the cell cycle. The delay of 3–5 weeks before viral gene expression is detectable would then reflect the time for the stem cell to enter G_1 (the first phase of mitosis), divide and for the daughter cells to move and enter the proliferative compartment of the epithelium (which includes both basal and parabasal cells), a population of cells permissive for viral gene expression.

Another phenomenon observed in COPV experimental infection supports this. Thus, if COPV is injected intra-dermally rather than applied by scarification the lag period is significantly extended by 2–3 weeks. This delay is particularly marked with low doses of infectious virus. Little epithelial wounding is associated with injection as compared to scarification and, therefore, little stimulus for epithelial wound healing during which keratinocyte stem cells transiently increase their replication rate. A dose effect might be expected if it is assumed that, at low doses, only a few stem cells in a given area are infected. In the absence of trauma these cells are recruited into cycle less frequently, with a resulting increase in the length of the lag phase.

Viral latency

Dependence upon the stem cell milieu for infection and immediate early viral gene expression would also partly explain the phenomenon of latency. HPV is frequently present as a latent infection in the female genital tract and the frequent lesion recurrence observed in respiratory papillomatosis is generally believed to reflect reactivation of latent infection rather than reinfection.[9] This is supported by the observation that histologically normal but HPV-positive laryngeal tissues express low-abundance transcripts coding for E1 and E2.[10] Similarly, in the rabbit low doses of CRPV lead to viral persistence and expression of truncated E1 and E2 transcripts but no lesion unless and until reactivation is induced by skin irritation. Furthermore, CRPV can persist at the site of regressed papillomas in 60% of cases with occasional lesion recurrence and similar phenomena are seen in bovine papillomavirus and COPV infections.[11] Latency is a poorly understood aspect of papillomavirus biology, but clearly of importance for therapeutic and prophylactic intervention strategies.

References

1. Walboomers JM, Jacobs MV, Manos MM *et al*. Human papillomavirus is a necessary cause of invasive cervical cancer worldwide. *J Pathol* 1999; **189**: 12–19.
2. Van Ranst M, Kaplan JB, Burk RD. Phylogenetic classification of human papillomaviruses: correlation with clinical manifestations. *J Gen Virol* 1992; **73**: 2653–60.
3. Kreider JW, Howett MK, Wolfe SA *et al*. Morphological transformation *in vivo* of human uterine cervix with papillomavirus from condylomata acuminata. *Nature* 1985; **317**: 639–41.

4. Stoler MH, Whitbeck A, Wolinsky SM *et al*. Infectious cycle of human papillomavirus type 11 in human foreskin xenografts in nude mice. *J Virol* 1990; **64**: 3310–18.

5. Nicholls PK, Klaunberg BA, Moore RA *et al*. Naturally occurring, nonregressing canine oral papillomavirus infection: host immunity, virus characterization, and experimental infection. *Virology* 1999; **265**: 365–74.

6. Zur Hausen H. Papillomaviruses and cancer: from basic studies to clinical application. *Nat Rev Cancer* 2002; **2**: 342–50.

7. Schmitt A, Rochat A, Zeltner R *et al*. The primary target cells of the high-risk cottontail rabbit papillomavirus colocalize with hair follicle stem cells. *J Virol* 1996; **70**: 1912–22.

8. Oriel JD. Natural history of genital warts. *Br J Venereal Diseases* 1971; **47**: 1–13.

9. Abramson AL, Steinberg BM, Winkler B. Laryngeal papillomatosis: clinical, histopathologic and molecular studies. *Laryngoscope* 1987; **97**: 678–85.

10. Maran A, Amella CA, Di Lorenzo TP *et al*. Human papillomavirus type 11 transcripts are present at low abundance in latently infected respiratory tissues. *Virology* 1995; **212**: 285–94.

11. Moore RA, Nicholls PK, Santos EB, Gough GW, Stanley MA. COPV DNA absence following prophylactic L1 PMID vaccination. *J Gen Virol* 2002; **83**: 2299–301.

Chapter 3
Immunology of the papillomaviruses

Margaret Stanley

Immune responses to virus infections

Before discussing papillomavirus-specific immunity it is helpful to review very briefly the basic features of the immune response to viruses. Put simply, cell-mediated immune responses are essential for the clearance of virus-infected cells and antibody-mediated humoral immunity clears free virus particles from body fluids and can prevent reinfection by virus.

T lymphocytes are the key players in cell-mediated immunity. T cells cannot recognize macromolecules, but need antigen processed into short peptides that are then bound to major histocompatibility complex (MHC) proteins and presented as a membrane-bound receptor complex on the cell surface. Polymorphic MHC molecules fall into two groups, human leukocyte antigen (HLA) class II (HLA-DP, HLA-DQ and HLA-DR) and class I (HLA-A, HLA-B and HLA-C). A class I MHC is expressed to varying extents on all cells except red cells, but class II is constitutively expressed only on professional antigen-presenting cells (APCs), i.e. dendritic cells, Langerhans' cells and B cells. There are two major subsets of T cells, CD8 and CD4 cells. CD4 cells recognize antigen together with class II MHCs, whereas CD8 cells recognize antigen together with class I MHCs. Usually an antigen plus a class II MHC is an exogenous antigen taken up from the extracellular milieu and broken down in the endosome of the APC for association into the class II complex for presentation on the cell surface and recognition by the specific T cell receptor on the CD4 T cell.

The interaction between the CD4 T cell and the APC is very complex requiring several other receptor–ligand interactions to occur in a regulated order before the T cell is activated and starts to proliferate. In particular, the T cell must receive a specific second signal from co-stimulatory molecules on the APC. Failure to receive the second signal can render the T cell anergic or unresponsive to any subsequent encounter with the antigen.

An antigen in the context of a class I MHC is an endogenous antigen derived usually but not always from intracellular synthesis of proteins broken down in the proteasome into short peptides and presented on the cell surface as an MHC–peptide complex for recognition by the T cell receptor on the CD8 lymphocyte. The geometry of the MHC–peptide complex is so precise that it is only recognized and bound with the correct affinity by a T cell receptor that matches it precisely.

T cell activation results in the secretion of a repertoire of small proteins or cytokines that help and regulate other cells. The pattern of cytokine expression defines two subsets of CD4 T cells

1. T helper 1 (Th1) cells secreting interferon-γ (IFN-γ) that help activate macrophages, natural killer (NK) cells and cytotoxic T lymphocytes (CTLs), thereby generating cell-mediated immunity.

2. T helper 2 (Th2) cells secreting interleukin-4 (IL-4) and IL-10 (and other cytokines) that help antigen-primed B lymphocytes in differentiating into plasma cells and secreting antibody for humoral responses (see Table 3.1).

Whether the CD4 T cell takes the Th2 or Th1 path is in turn very strongly influenced by the APC as a consequence of the receptors it expresses and the cytokines secreted. These functions of the APC are in turn activated by signals received from other receptor–ligand interactions (in particular toll-like receptors on the APC) between it and the pathogen. The APC in effect 'tells' the T cell what sort of defence is needed and is central to the generation of an effective and appropriate immune response (Figure 3.1).

It seems that only professional APCs can initiate primary immune responses and activate virgin T cells, but human papil-

Response	Characteristics
Type 1/Th1: cell mediated	Class II MHC-restricted CD4 T lymphocytes secreting IFN-γ Effectors are class I MHC-restricted CD8 cells, NK cells, activated macrophages and cytotoxic antibodies
Type 2/Th2: humoral	Class II MHC-restricted CD4 T lymphocytes secreting IL-4 Help antigen-primed B cells in differentiating and secreting non-cytotoxic antibodies as effectors

Table 3.1
Adaptive immune responses

lomavirus (HPV) proteins are only expressed in keratinocytes so how can cell-mediated immune responses be induced against them? There are various scenarios. Dendritic cells, via their dendritic process, constantly sample the surfaces of their cellular neighbours phagocytosing fragments released from them. Antigen released from dying cells is taken up by the APC and enters both the class I and class II processing pathways. HPV proteins could be accessed in this way and, in this situation, the APC first presents processed peptide to the CD4 T cell. The T cell then signals back to the APC via CD40–CD40 ligand interactions. This activates or licenses the APC to present directly to naive CD8 T cells that can then differentiate into potent CTLs that will search out and kill HPV-infected cells expressing the same viral peptide–MHC I complex presented to them originally by the APC (Figure 3.2).

Immune responses to papillomavirus infection

The infectious cycle of the papillomaviruses raises several important questions with respect to immune recognition. These are not acute infections: an interval of at least 6 weeks elapses between infection and the release of new infectious virus (because this time interval is required for the completion of the keratinocyte differentiation programme). Virus replication and release of infectious virus does not induce inflammation and, as a result, there is no 'danger signal' for alerting the immune system to virus activity. The papillomaviruses have a strategy that results in persistent chronic infections, as the host remains ignorant of the pathogen for long periods. So is there an immune response and, if there is, what does it consist of and how and where is it evoked?

*Figure 3.1
Activation of naive
CD4+ T lymphocytes.
The CD 4+ T cell
with a T cell receptor
that recognizes and
binds perfectly to the
class II MHC–peptide
complex displayed
on the surface of
the dendritic cell
can be activated to
proliferate provided
it receives a second
molecular signal,
via molecules such
as CD80, from the
dendritic cell. The
activated cells can
differentiate down the
Th1 or Th2 pathway.
This decision depends
significantly on the
cytokine environment
generated by the
dendritic cell and this
in turn depends upon
signals received by the
dendritic cell from the
pathogen recognition
receptors that it
bears. Members of
the toll-like receptor
family are important
pathogen recognition
receptors and some
members can bias the
differentiation down
the Th1 pathway
by stimulating the
dendritic cell to
secrete IL-12 and type
I interferons.*

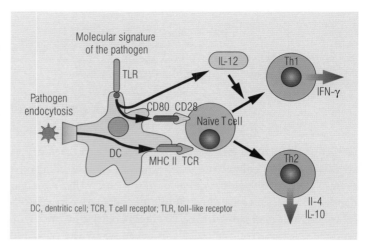

Cell-mediated immunity in human papillomavirus infections

The increased incidence and progression of HPV infections in immunosuppressed individuals illustrates the critical role of cell-mediated immune responses in the resolution and control of HPV infections.[1] Human immunodeficiency virus (HIV)-infected patients show multiple recurrences of cervical HPV infections and an increased incidence of genital warts that appears to reflect an increased risk of progression from subclinical to clinical infection. The evidence from allograft recipients and HIV-infected individuals indicates that it is the absolute deficit in CD4 T cells that is the important risk factor for HPV-induced disease and associated neoplastic progression in the immunocompromised individual. This suggests that CD4 T cells play a central role in the resolution and control of HPV infection.

Histological studies

Clues as to the nature of the cellular immune response to HPV infection have come from immunohistological studies of spontaneously regressing genital warts.[2] Non-regressing genital warts are characterized by a lack of immune cells, the few

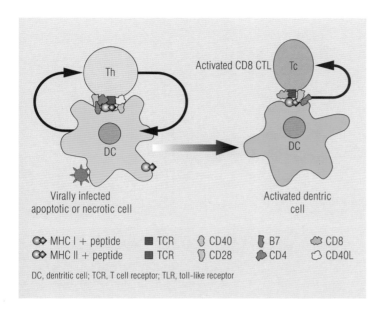

Th

Activated CD8 CTL   Tc

DC

DC

Virally infected
apoptotic or necrotic cell

Activated dentric
cell

◐ MHC I + peptide   ■ TCR   ◊ CD40   ß B7   ⬠ CD8
◐ MHC II + peptide   ■ TCR   ◊ CD28   ◆ CD4   ○ CD40L

DC, dentritic cell; TCR, T cell receptor; TLR, toll-like receptor

Figure 3.2
CD4+ T cells can help generate CD8+ killer T cells. HPVs do not infect antigen-presenting cells and it is probable that HPV early proteins released from infected cells are captured by a dendritic cell, processed and presented to naive CD4+ cells as described before. This interaction results in a signal back to the dendritic cell that is then able to present peptides associated with class I MHC effectively to the naive CD 8+ T cell with the generation of HPV antigen-specific cytotoxic T cells that will bind to and kill any cell expressing the class I MHC–peptide complex against which they were activated by the dendritic cell. DC, dendritic cell; TCR, T cell receptor.

intra-epithelial lymphocytes are CD8 cells and mononuclear cells are present mainly in the stroma. When warts regress there is a massive mononuclear cell infiltrate in both the stroma and epithelium. CD4 cells dominate this, but many CD8 cells are present (Figure 3.3). The infiltrating lymphocytes are activated and express surface markers that show that they are 'antigen-experienced' or memory cells. The wart keratinocytes express class II MHCs and there is up-regulation of the adhesion molecules required for lymphocyte trafficking on the endothelium of the wart capillaries. These appearances are characteristic of a Th1-biased lymphocyte response and the release of Th1-type cytokines such as IFN-γ and IL-12. Analysis of cytokine expression in regressing warts confirms the morphological evidence for a Th1 response in the regressing lesions with expression of mRNA for the pro-inflammatory cytokines IFN-γ, tumour necrosis factor-α (TNF-α) and IL-12. Interestingly, bioactive IL-12 is expressed not only by dendritic cells and macrophages in the regressing wart, but also by the infected keratinocytes.

Figure 3.3 Spontaneous regression in anogenital warts is characterized by (a) an intense mononuclear cell infiltrate composed of both (b) CD4+ T cells and (c) CD8+ T cells.

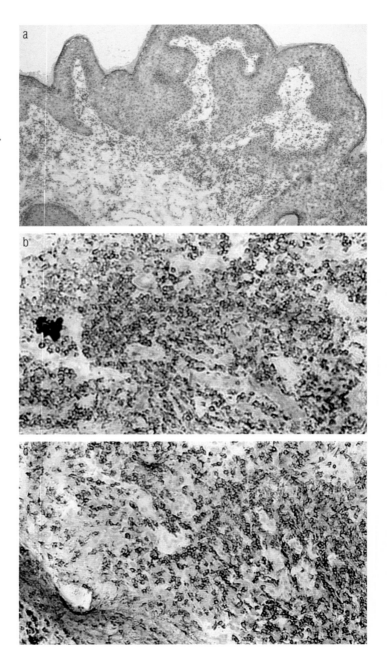

Immune events in regressing canine oral papillomavirus infections

Cross-sectional studies can only provide a snapshot of what is a dynamic process. Longitudinal studies in patients are logistically difficult and animal models of mucosal papillomavirus infection, such as canine oral papillomavirus (COPV), are needed if the immunological events of the entire wart cycle from infection to regression are to be followed. At the present time COPV is the best animal model for mucosatrophic papillomavirus infection. The lesions are similar to those induced by the genital mucosatrophic viruses, but contain large amounts of infectious virus. After infection by abrasion of the mucosal surface, oral papillomas are generated within 6–8 weeks, before regressing spontaneously within 12–16 weeks, after which the animals are immune to challenge with infectious virus.

The immune events accompanying COPV-induced wart regression are shown in Figure 3.4. Regression is preceded at weeks 7–8 post-infection by emigration from the lesion of Langerhans' cells and migration into the stroma of CD4+ T cells, principally $\alpha\beta$ T cells, followed by a smaller subset of CD8+ T cells. CD8+ cells reach a peak just as the wart completes regression at weeks 9–10 post-infection. Numerous apoptotic keratinocytes are demonstrable in regressing lesions and it appears that keratinocyte apoptosis may play an important role in lesion regression since it correlates both spatially and temporally with lymphocyte infiltration and wart regression. COPV L1 capsid protein is detectable in the lesions at week 7 reaching a maximum at week 8. At week 8 neutralizing antibody to the major capsid protein L1 is just detectable, but by weeks 11–12 there is a marked increase in titre. In the subsequent weeks antibody levels decline slowly but are still detectable at 12–18 months post-infection. The immunohistological events accompanying wart regression in COPV infection parallel the changes seen in clinical biopsies of regressing genital warts very closely (Figure 3.2). However, all animals undergo seroconversion post-wart clearance, a phenomenon that does not apply to humans clearing ano-genital warts.[3]

Figure 3.4
The regression of
COPV-infected
warts is mediated
via CD4 and
CD8 cells that
infiltrate the wart
at week 7 just
before regression
starts at week
8. Neutralizing
antibody to the
L1 capsid protein
is not detectable
until the regression
is complete and
peaks at that time.
Antibody levels
decline slowly over
the subsequent
weeks but low
levels remain for
several months.
The regression does
not result in the
clearance of viral
DNA and the virus
remains in a latent
state probably
for the lifetime
of the animal.
Wart recurrence is
almost unknown
unless the animal is
immunosuppressed.

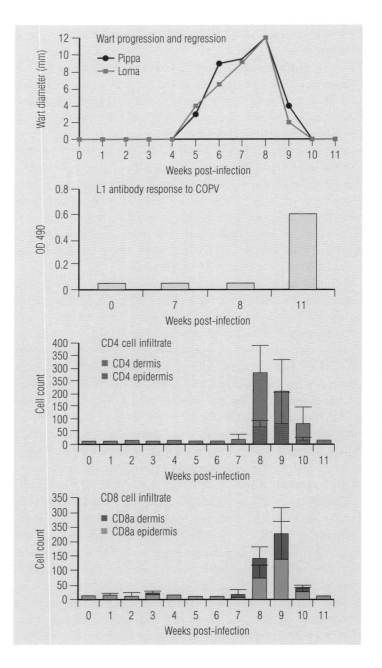

T cell responses in human papillomavirus infections

Methods for measuring cell-mediated immunity

Cell-mediated immune responses to viral antigens are usually assayed using peripheral blood mononuclear cells (PBMCs). Helper T cell responses to antigen are often measured by lymphoproliferation assays in which PBMCs are incubated with antigen (usually in the form of protein or peptides) for varying periods of time, at the end of which the proliferative capacity of the cells is measured by ^{3}H-thymidine uptake. Assay of cytokine release from antigen-stimulated T cells can also be used. CTL assays have until recently depended upon measurement of the cytotoxicity of antigen against ^{51}Cr-labelled target cells, which is a laborious and relatively insensitive method since only cells able to survive and proliferate *in vitro* can be assayed. New methods overcome this and allow direct analysis of antigen-specific T cells from the blood without the necessity for lengthy *in vitro* manipulations. Enzyme-linked immunospot assays that measure the number of cells secreting key cytokines, e.g. IFN-γ or IL-5, are now commonly used and, when combined with methods for separating T cell subsets so that, for example, either CD4+ or CD8+ cells are analysed, increase the sensitivity and specificity.

It is important to recognize the limitations of these methods when applied to determining responses to HPV antigens. The use of appropriate controls is essential. Positive controls are necessary for checking that the PBMCs are functional and react to test antigens and negative controls are essential for confirming that the assay conditions used are supporting only HPV-specific T cell responses. A problem for HPV studies is identifying true negative controls since HPV infections are common and may be subclinical or latent. Another difficulty is that viral proteins must be generated by recombinant expression technologies and then purified. The controls must therefore always include expression system products (bacterial proteins or protein tags for example) that could be immunogenic. Overall, the cleanest data have been obtained by using panels of synthetic peptides overlapping in sequence.

CD4 T cell responses

Immunohistological studies have clearly indicated that regression of HPV-infected lesions is associated with a Th1 response, but the viral antigens that provoke this response still remain to be identified unequivocally. The evidence from both experimental models and human studies shows that viral proteins are immune targets. Delayed-type hypersensitivity (DTH) responses to the early genes E6 and E7 can be shown in a murine model in which viral antigen is expressed in keratinocytes and mimics the natural route of infection. The ability for priming the immune system and eliciting a DTH response in this system depends upon antigen dose.[4] Low levels of antigen induce immune non-responsiveness, which is a phenomenon associated with a switch in Th1–Th2 cytokine expression in the CD8 subset in the draining lymph node that is suggestive of a suppresser effect.

Most studies have concentrated on responses to high-risk HPV E6 and E7 proteins or the L1 capsid protein in patients with cervical HPV-associated disease. Specific T cell responses to HPV 16 E7 and L1 have been identified in patients with cervical intra-epithelial neoplasia (CIN) of various grades in cross-sectional studies. Overall, these studies show that CD4+ responses to L1 are common in HPV-infected patients, but are also detected in controls. T cell responses to E7 are more common in high-grade than low-grade cervical intra-epithelial disease, but decline significantly in carcinoma patients. Those with high-grade lesions contained a higher proportion of responders than the CIN grade 1 group. T cell-proliferative responses to HPV 16 E7 were described in a longitudinal study in which patients fell into three groups: those who cleared disease, those with persistent disease and those with progressive disease.[5] Interestingly, the strongest T cell responses were observed in women with persisting HPV infection and progressing cervical lesions (99% reactive) compared to those with clearing or fluctuating infection (41% reactive). A different outcome was reported in a study by Kadish et al.[6] who determined T cell-proliferative responses to E6 and E7 peptides at intervals of 3 months over a period of 12 months in a cohort of women with CIN I or II. The cell-mediated immune responses in this group to a specific E7 peptide correlated significantly with the regression of disease and resolution of infection.[6] Intriguingly these responses were not HPV type specific.

There are interesting recent data on CD4+ T cell responses to HPV 11 L1 virus-like particles (VLPs) in 25 healthy adults.[7] Remarkably 80% of these subjects were responders in that HPV 11 L1-specific CD4+ T cell lines could be established from the memory T cell subset that expresses the CD45 RO surface marker. This high frequency of T cell responses contrasts with the prevalence of the antibody response to HPV 11 in the general population, which is of the order of 12%. Interestingly, in this study there was marked cross-reactivity with other HPV types, a phenomenon also described in individuals vaccinated with HPV 11 VLPs in a phase II prophylactic vaccine trial.[8] Antibody responses to HPV VLPs are type specific and the significance of these promiscuous T cell responses to L1 with respect to vaccine strategies remains to be established.

T cell responses to early antigens other than E6 and E7 have not been well documented. However, there is increasing evidence that the E2 protein is an important immune target for effective viral clearance. In cottontail rabbit virus (CRPV) infection in the rabbit, which provides a good model for papilloma/carcinoma progression, the induction of T cell-proliferative responses to E2 protein was the best predictor of lesion regression.[9] In a recent study HPV 16 E2-specific Th responses could be detected in 50% of healthy donors suggesting that E2-specific CD4+ memory is associated with a successful host response to HPV infection.[10]

Few studies have determined the antigen specificity of lymphocytes infiltrating HPV-infected lesions. Hong et al.[11]

isolated wart-infiltrating lymphocytes from HPV 6-infected ano-genital warts and characterized their response to HPV 6 E7 and L1 proteins in a lymphoproliferation assay. HPV 6 E7- or L1-specific wart-infiltrating lymphocytes could be isolated from more than 75% of the patients studied ($n = 24$). Interestingly, despite the huge variation between patients in surface markers of the wart-infiltrating lymphocytes (CD4, CD8, T cell receptor $\alpha\beta$ or T cell receptor $\gamma\delta$), the HPV 6 E7 and L1 peptides recognized by wart-infiltrating lymphocytes differed from those recognized by peripheral T cells. No CTL activity against L1 or E7 could be demonstrated in this study and, since the warts were surgically excised, whether these lesions would have persisted or regressed is not known.

Cytotoxic T cell responses

The role of CTLs in HPV infection is a topic of intense contemporary interest and again studies have concentrated on responses to HPV 16 E6 and E7 proteins in cervical HPV-associated disease. HPV-specific CTLs can be detected in patients with previous or ongoing HPV infection. Natural history studies will be the most informative here and Nakagawa *et al.*[12] reported on a small group of patients, nine with cleared HPV infection and 11 with newly diagnosed HPV 16-positive CIN. CTL responses were identified in both groups, but those who cleared infection were more frequent responders (63%) than those with current CIN (14%) implying that an effective CTL response is important for the clearance of infection.[12] Both CD4 and CD8 cytotoxic effectors have been shown to be involved in these responses. CTL responses have been shown in patients with grade 3 CIN and cervical carcinoma, but not in normal controls in cross-sectional studies.[13] Recent studies using a highly sensitive assay whereby fluorescently labelled HLA–peptide complexes (tetramers) are detected show that high-affinity HPV E7-specific CTLs are rare but detectable in patients with carcinoma or high-grade CIN.[14] The association between HPV 16 E6- and E7-specific CTLs and HPV 16 persistence was examined in a longitudinal study of women with polymerase chain reaction-determined cervical HPV 16 infection. Lack of a CTL response to E6 but not E7 correlated with persistent HPV infection, thereby suggesting that a CTL response to HPV 16 E6 is important for viral clearance and, by implication, neoplastic progression.[15]

Cytotoxic effector mechanisms also include NK cells, a subset of lymphocytes that kill virally infected or tumour cells lacking surface expression of class I MHC molecules, the so-called 'altered self' hypothesis. NK cells appear to be required for the clearance of only certain viruses and these appear to include HPV. There is evidence for defective NK cell function in HPV 16-associated disease in that PBMCs from patients with active HPV 16 neoplastic disease display a reduced NK cell activity against HPV 16-infected keratinocytes. In vitro expression of the E7 protein of HPV 16/18 precludes the lysis of HPV-transformed cells by IFN-stimulated NK cells and the E6/E7 proteins of HPV 16 inhibit IL-18 expression by NK cells by binding to both IL-18 and its receptor.[16] IFN-α is an important activator of resting NK cells and HPV 16 E6 and E7 proteins can inhibit the induction of IFN-α-inducible genes. Target recognition by NK cells does not involve classical antigen receptors because these cells do not express T or B cell antigen receptors, nor do they rearrange their immunoglobulin or T cell receptor genes. This apparent lack of antigen-specific receptors and MHC recognition originally led to the view that NK cell-mediated killing was broad and non-MHC restricted, but it turns out that NK cells express clonally distributed receptors specific for class I MHC-type molecules that can be functionally inhibitory or stimulatory. Inhibitory receptors block NK cell-mediated cytotoxicity upon binding to HLA ligands. Stimulatory receptors also bind HLA class I motifs but trigger NK cell-mediated cytotoxicity. NK cell-mediated cytolysis of a virally infected or tumour cell depends upon the balance between the negative and positive signals received by the NK cell. It is evident that the expression of these molecules and class I MHC expression is critical for cytotoxic effector mechanisms and loss of or down-regulation of them would be a way whereby viruses such as HPV evade host defences.

Immunogenetics and human papillomavirus infection

The HLA haplotype of the individual could influence the natural history of HPV infection in that individual since, for any one protein antigen, different alleles of the MHC will present different peptides to the immune system. Thus, the HLA haplotype of the individual could be a major determinant of whether infection is cleared or persists which, in the case of the oncogenic viruses, could influence the risk of neoplastic progression. If this thesis is correct then it could be reflected in different HLA frequencies in patients with persistent or chronic HPV infections compared to the appropriate control populations.

Data from the rabbit strongly support this supposition since the regression or progression of papillomas induced by CRPV is strongly linked to the MHC DR or DQ phenotypes of the animals, respectively.[17] Recurrent respiratory papillomatosis represents an extreme form of persistent HPV infection and overrepresentation of HLA-DQ3 and DQ11 alleles has been reported in these patients.[18] A number of studies have examined associations between HLA haplotype and cervical carcinoma, but the evidence is that the associations are between HPV type and HLA. This was first raised in a case–control study of Hispanic women with cervical cancer compared to those with normal Pap smears from the South West USA. It was found that certain HLA class II haplotypes including DRB1*150–DQB1*0602 were significantly associated with HPV 16-containing cancer, whereas DR13 haplotypes were negatively associated.[19] The association of susceptibility to HPV 16 infection and these haplotypes has been shown in other well-controlled studies and, importantly, such individuals tend to have more long-term infections. Host genetic factors such as variation at the class II locus will influence host responses to the virus and the outcome of infection.

Humoral immunity

The role of the humoral immune response in HPV infections has been clarified recently. It is clear that antibodies have little to do with the maintenance of infection since disorders of humoral immunity do not result in increased susceptibility to HPV. However, natural infections in animals, such as the rabbit and cow, show that antibodies against the major capsid protein L1 are protective. Studies on humoral immunity to HPV, particularly to the high-risk genital HPVs, have been seriously hampered by the lack of suitable antigenic targets for serological assays since neither clinical lesions nor *in vitro* culture systems are practical sources of virus. These problems have been solved by the demonstration that expression of the L1 capsid protein via recombinant vectors results in the self-assembly of the protein into a conformationally correct VLP.[20,21] Numerous sero-epidemiological studies have been undertaken using HPV VLPs as the antigen in enzyme-linked immunosorbent assays (ELISAs). Overall, the evidence from studies on both the high- and low-risk genital viruses is that specific antibody responses to the L1 capsid protein as measured in the VLP ELISA are common during and after infection with genital HPVs. However, the low sensitivity of the assay and the variability of the interval between infection and seroconversion suggest that serum antibody responses are not useful for diagnosis in the individual patient, but are of value as markers of past or current HPV infection in population-based studies.

Antibody reactivity to early proteins has been examined in several studies. There is good evidence for antibody reactivity to the early proteins E6 and E7 in patients with cervical carcinoma although there is no evidence that this has prognostic significance.[22] Seroreactivity to the immunodominant region of HPV 16 E7 was examined using a peptide-based ELISA in a longitudinal cohort study of women all presenting initially with HPV-positive mild to moderate dyskaryosis. During follow-up the cohort divided into those who cleared the infection, those who had fluctuating infection and those who had persistent infection. The highest titres and the highest numbers of responders were found in those who cleared the infection, but patients with persistent infection were more consistently seronegative.[23]

Interestingly, analysis of the immunoglobulin G (IgG) subclass showed that IgG_2 was dominant in patients who cleared infection whereas IgG_1 and IgG_2 were produced equally in patients with frank invasive carcinoma, thereby suggesting that clearance was associated with a cell-mediated or Th1 response but that progression involved a shift to a Th2 response. Responses to the E2 protein of the high-risk viruses have been reported in several studies, although the significance of these studies, many of which were peptide based, is difficult to assess. A relationship between serum IgA anti-E2 antibodies and the stage and progression of cervical neoplasia was shown in a study using a baculovirus-derived protein in a radio-precipitation immunoassay with a decrease in IgA anti-E2 correlating with progression.[24]

Human papillomavirus vaccines

Looking at the evidence overall the following seems to be a reasonable scenario for the host response to HPV infection in the genital tract. Natural history studies have shown that genital HPV infection is common but most infections resolve without intervention. The evidence from animal models and regressing warts is that resolution is due to a Th1 response that is CD4 dependent, although the nature of the effectors is still not known unequivocally. Seroconversion and the generation of serum-neutralizing antibody to the major capsid protein L1 accompany a successful immune response in animal infections and probably in humans. Failure to induce an immune response seems to be due to inefficient priming: the immune system is effectively not 'told' that virus is present. Successful control or immunotherapies for these infections will either prevent infection and/or induce a strong virus-specific Th1 response for the clearance of established infections and indeed both prophylactic and therapeutic vaccines against HPV infections are either under clinical trial or in advanced pre-clinical development.

Prophylactic vaccines

Prophylactic vaccines will generate neutralizing antibody to viral capsid proteins and VLPs are obvious candidate immunogens for this. Overall the data from published phase I studies using HPV VLP vaccines, including HPV 16/18[25] or and/or HPV 6/11 L1 VLPs,[8] show that these vaccines are safe, well tolerated and highly immunogenic, inducing high levels of both binding- and neutralizing-type antibodies and phase II and phase III trials are in progress with these vaccines. In at least one of the phase III studies, vaccine efficacy will be measured as prevention of the persistence of HPV DNA and the development of both low- and high-grade squamous intra-epithelial lesions. The key issues are whether the antibodies generated will be protective, how long the protection will last and to what extent they will be cross-protective against infection with other types. Early data from proof of principle efficacy trials for HPV 16 have indicated that the antibodies generated are protective, but there is no information as yet on the duration of protection and cross-reactivity.[26]

The data emerging from the HPV VLP vaccine trials are immensely encouraging, but there are concerns relating more to social and economic issues rather than scientific ones. The major burden of malignant HPV-associated disease is in women in the developing world. Vaccines for these women must be cheap and easily delivered. VLP vaccines are likely to be expensive and require medical or paramedical personnel for delivery and cold storage for maintaining stability. It is unlikely that they will be the optimal vaccine for the developing world, but will be widely taken up in developed countries. Cheap and easily delivered alternatives are required. DNA vaccines may fill this niche, but still have problems of delivery. Vaccines delivered directly to mucosal surfaces such as the oral or intra-nasal surface could be relatively inexpensive and this may be an area where HPV genes expressed in plants provide a cheap source. However, the reality of prophylactic vaccination via the mucosal route for HPV remains to be demonstrated

Therapeutic vaccines

The induction of strong cell-mediated immune responses is central to any therapeutic vaccine strategy and may be critical for long-term immunity in prophylaxis. HPV early proteins do not evoke strong immune responses during the natural infection, but there is a strong body of evidence from animal models that deliberate immunization with them may be an effective therapeutic strategy. It was shown several years ago that immunization in the CRPV model with the non-structural proteins E1 and E2 induced a strong T cell response and enhanced the regression of papillomas.[27] Recent data from the COPV model using DNA vaccines support this and suggest further that a key determinant of vaccine efficacy is the antigen expression level. Papillomavirus genes express at relatively low levels in mammalian cells even when under the control of strong heterologous promoters since codon usage is not optimal. A polynucleotide vaccine comprising a codon-modified COPV E2 gene delivered by gene gun prevented papilloma formation in dogs previously challenged with COPV (R.A. Moore, personal communication). These data from animal models have significant implications for the design of HPV vaccines. They suggest that the early proteins to be included in vaccines for the prevention of infection or treatment of low-grade or benign HPV-associated disease should at least include E2 and that the level of antigen expression will be crucial. Such vaccines are likely to be combined with immunomodulators such as cytokines or immune response modifiers such as imiquimod in order to maximize the response.

Therapeutic vaccination strategies for HPV-associated ano-genital malignancies have a relatively simple rationale. In cervical cancers and probably most high-grade pre-cancers viral gene regulation is deregulated and the E6 and E7 genes are constitutively expressed. The continued expression of these oncogenes is essential for progression to and maintenance of the malignant phenotype. Since these viral proteins are expressed specifically by the tumour cells then peptide fragments will be displayed in association with a class I MHC on the cell surface and be targets for CTL killing. Hence, the generation of HPV 16 E6 and/or E7 CTLs by deliberate immunization should be an effective therapy in HPV-associated high-grade intra-epithelial lesions and cancer. However, immunotherapies for HPV-associated high-grade pre-cancers and invasive cancers are problematic. Tumour evasion mechanisms, such as down-regulation of a class I MHC that removes the CTL target, remain a tough barrier for successful cancer immunotherapies.

Summary of immune responses

HPV infection in the genital tract is common in young, sexually active individuals, the majority of whom clear the infection without overt clinical disease. Those who develop lesions in most cases also mount an effective cell-mediated immune response and the lesions regress. Lesions in which productive viral infection is occurring (ano-genital warts and CIN I) are not associated with inflammation or histological evidence of immune activity. The regression of ano-genital warts is accompanied histologically by a response characteristic of DTH: animal models support this and provide evidence that the response is regulated by CD4 T cell-dependent mechanisms. The increased prevalence of HPV infections in individuals who are immunosuppressed either as a consequence of organ transplantation or HIV infection demonstrates the central importance of the CD4 T cell population in the control of established HPV infections. Although it seems clear that the CD4 T cell subset is critical for the induction and regulation of the host response to HPV the nature of the effector response remains unclear. There is increasing evidence that both NK cells and antigen-specific CTLs are important effectors, but these responses are still poorly understood.

Antibody responses to the major virus capsid protein L1 accompany the induction of successful cell-mediated immunity and these responses are certainly protective against subsequent viral challenge in natural infections in animals, thereby suggesting that prophylactic immunization will be effective in controlling HPV-induced genital disease. If the cell-mediated response fails to induce lesion regression and viral clearance then a persistent viral infection results, which is in part due to operational immune tolerance. This seems to be reflected by the *in vitro* detection of enhanced cellular and humoral responses to early viral proteins and the failure of these responses to clear virus *in vivo*. The importance of the MHC in susceptibility to or protection from papillomavirus infection and disease remains a crucial one for investigation.

References

1. Benton EC, Arends MJ. Human papillomavirus in the immu-nosuppressed. In Lacey C (editor). *Papillomavirus Reviews: Current Research on Papillomaviruses*. Leeds: Leeds University Press; 1996: pp. 271–9.

2. Coleman N, Birley HD, Renton AM *et al*. Immunological events in regressing genital warts. *Am J Clin Pathol* 1994; **102**: 768–74.

3. Carter JJ, Wipf GC, Hagensee ME *et al*. Use of human papil-lomavirus type 6 capsids to detect antibodies in people with genital warts. *J Infect Dis* 1995; **172**: 11–18.

4. Chambers MA, Wei Z, Coleman N, Nash AA, Stanley MA. 'Natural' presentation of human papillomavirus type 16 E7 protein to immunocompetent mice results in antigen specific sensitization or sustained unresponsiveness. *Eur J Immunol* 1994; **24**: 738–45.

5. De Gruijl TD, Bontkes HJ, Walboomers JM *et al*. Analysis of IgG reactivity against human papillomavirus type-16 E7 in patients with cervical intraepithelial neoplasia indicates an asso-ciation with clearance of viral infection: results of a prospective study. *Int J Cancer* 1996; **68**: 731–8.

6. Kadish AS, Timmins P, Wang Y *et al*. Regression of cervical intraepithelial neoplasia and loss of human papillomavirus (HPV) infection is associated with cell-mediated immune responses to an HPV type 16 E7 peptide. *Cancer Epidemiol Biomarkers Prev* 2002; **11**: 483–8.

7. Williams OM, Hart KW, Wang ECY, Gelder CM. Analysis of CD4(+) T-cell responses to human papillomavirus (HPV) type 11 L1 in healthy adults reveals a high degree of responsiveness and cross-reactivity with other HPV types. *J Virol* 2002; **76**: 7418–29.

8. Evans TG, Bonnez W, Rose RC *et al*. A phase 1 study of a recom-binant viruslike particle vaccine against human papillomavirus type 11 in healthy adult volunteers. *J Infect Dis* 2001; **183**: 1485–93.

9. Selvakumar R, Borenstein LA, Lin Y-L, Ahmed R, Wettstein FO. Immunization with nonstructural proteins E1 and E2 of cotton tail rabbit papillomavirus stimulates regression of virus-induced papillomas. *J Virol* 1995; **69**: 602–5.

10. De Jong A, Van der Burg SH, Kwappenberg KMC *et al*. Frequent detection of human papillomavirus 16 E2-specific T-helper immunity in healthy subjects. *Cancer Res* 2002; **62**: 472–9.

11. Hong K, Greer CE, Ketter N, Van Nest G, Paliard X. Isolation and characterization of human papillomavirus type 6-specific T cells infiltrating genital warts. *J Virol* 1997; **71**: 6427–32.

12. Nakagawa M, Stites DP, Palefsky JM, Kneass Z, Moscicki AB. CD4-positive and CD8-positive cytotoxic T lymphocytes contribute to human papillomavirus type 16 E6 and E7 responses. *Clin Diagn Lab Immunol* 1999; **6**: 494–8.

13. Nimako M, Fiander AN, Wilkinson GWG, Borysiewicz LK, Man S. Human papillomavirus-specific cytotoxic T lymphocytes in patients with cervical intraepithelial neoplasia grade III. *J Virol* 1997; **57**: 4855–61.

14. Youde SJ, Dunbar PR, Evans EM *et al*. Use of fluorogenic histocompatibility leukocyte antigen-A*0201/HPV 16 E7 peptide complexes to isolate rare human cytotoxic T-lymphocyte-recognizing endogenous human papillomavirus antigens. *Cancer Res* 2000; **60**: 365–71.

15. Bontkes HJ, De Gruijl TD, Van den Muysenberg AJ *et al*. Human papillomavirus type 16 E6/E7-specific cytotoxic T lymphocytes in women with cervical neoplasia. *Int J Cancer* 2000; **88**: 92–8.

16. Lee SJ, Cho YS, Cho MC *et al*. Both E6 and E7 oncoproteins of human papillomavirus 16 inhibit IL-18-induced IFN-gamma production in human peripheral blood mononuclear and NK cells. *J Immunol* 2001; **167**: 497–504.

17. Han R, Breitburd F, Marche PN, Orth G. Linkage of regression and malignant conversion of rabbit viral papillomas to MHC class II genes [see comments]. *Nature* 1992; **356**: 66–8.

18. Bonagura VR, Siegal FP, Abramson AL *et al*. Enriched HLA DQ3 phenotype and decreased class I major histocompatibility complex antigen expression in recurrent respiratory papillomatosis. *Clin Diagn Lab Immunol* 1994; **1**: 357–60.

19. Apple RJ, Erlich HA, Klitz W *et al*. HLA DR DQ associations with cervical carcinoma show papillomavirus type specificity. *Nat Genet* 1994; **6**: 157–62.

20. Zhou J, Sun XY, Stenzel DJ, Frazer IH. Expression of vaccinia recombinant HPV 16 L1 and L2 ORF proteins in epithelial cells is sufficient for assembly of HPV virion like particles. *Virology* 1991; **185**: 251–7.

21. Kirnbauer R, Booy F, Cheng N, Lowy DR, Schiller JT. Papillomavirus L1 major capsid protein self assembles into virus like particles that are highly immunogenic. *Proc Natl Acad Sci USA* 1992; **89**: 12180–4.

22. Stacey SN, Ghosh A, Bartholomew JS *et al.* Expression of human papillomavirus type 16 E7 protein by recombinant baculovirus and use for the detection of E7 antibodies in sera from cervical carcinoma patients. *J Med Virol* 1993; **40**: 14–21.

23. De Gruijl TD, Bontkes HJ, Stukart MJ *et al.* T cell proliferative responses against human papillomavirus type 16 E7 oncoprotein are most prominent in cervical intraepithelial neoplasia patients with persistent viral infection. *J Gen Virol* 1996; **77**: 2183–91.

24. Rocha Zavaleta L, Jordan D, Pepper S *et al.* Differences in serological IgA responses to recombinant baculovirus-derived human papillomavirus E2 protein in the natural history of cervical neoplasia. *Br J Cancer* 1997; **75**: 1144–50.

25. Harro CD, Pang YY, Roden RB *et al.* Safety and immunogenicity trial in adult volunteers of a human papillomavirus 16 L1 virus-like particle vaccine. *J Natl Cancer Inst* 2001; **93**: 284–92.

26. Koutsky LA, Ault KA, Wheeler CM *et al.* A controlled trial of a human papillomavirus type 16 vaccine. *N Engl J Med* 2002; **347**: 1645–51.

27. Selvakumar R, Ahmed R, Wettstein FO. Tumor regression is associated with a specific immune response to the E2 protein of cotton tail rabbit papillomavirus. *Virology* 1995; **208**: 298–302.

Chapter 4
Treatments

Jane Sterling

Introduction

Many different methods of treatment are available for genital
warts. Unfortunately, none gives a 100% chance of clearance
or a 0% chance of recurrence, which would be the ideal. The
choice of therapy depends on many factors, such as operator
experience and the age, sensitivity or preference of the patient.
In all cases the perfect treatment would be well tolerated and
produce little skin damage and no long-term scarring.

Topical preparations are likely to penetrate the soft
non-keratinized surfaces of mucosal warts in comparison
with areas of hard keratinized warts. However, increased
penetration usually also means increased local side effects,
particularly those of inflammation, which are very common
with many commonly used wart therapies.

In the absence of a specific anti-viral therapy, the aims of
genital wart treatments are to reverse the changes that are
occurring within the abnormal epithelium and to encourage
an immune response to the virally infected cells. Different
treatments have different effects including (1) reduction of
growth of the epidermis, (2) direct destruction of the abnormal
tissue and (3) stimulation of immune activity at the site of the
wart (Table 4.1). Warts can clear naturally by normal immune
responses. Using data from several trials in which a placebo
treatment has been used it is estimated that up to 20% of patients
may clear their warts spontaneously within approximately
3 months.

Table 3.1
The differing effects
and applications
of genital wart
treatments

Mechanism of action	Method of use	Therapy
Anti-proliferation	Topical	Podophyllin
		Podophyllotoxin
		5-FU*
		Cidofovir*
	Systemic	Retinoid*
Destructive	Topical	Monochloroacetic acid
		Trichloroacetic acid
	Intra-lesional	Bleomycin*
		Photodynamic therapy*
	Surgical	Cryotherapy
		Excision etc.
Immune stimulation	Topical	Imiquimod
	Intra-lesional	IFN*
	Systemic	IFN*
		Cimetidine*
		Therapeutic vaccination*

*Treatments not used in routine practice and may not be of proven benefit.

Anti-proliferative therapies

Podophyllin

Podophyllin resin is extracted from the roots of the May apple plant. It contains several different compounds and the relative strengths of these compounds are variable depending on the extraction. The podophyllin resin is used in a 10–25% solution in benzoin tincture (tincture of benzoin compound) for application to the skin.

The main active ingredient of podophyllin resin for the treatment of warts is podophyllotoxin. Podophyllotoxin acts as an anti-mitotic agent, interfering with cell division by disrupting the formation of the mitotic spindle on which chromosomes distribute before the cell divides. It therefore damages tissues in which cells are reproducing.

Method of treatment

The usual method of treatment with podophyllin is a weekly or twice weekly application in the clinic by a doctor or nurse. The preparation of podophyllin is used at a strength of 15–25% in benzoin tincture and is applied by a small cotton wool bud to the surface of the wart(s) and immediately surrounding skin. The application should dry before the patient dresses and must be washed off after 4–8 h. The treatment is usually repeated for 4 or 5 weeks. Home treatment by the patient with these preparations is not recommended as over-enthusiastic use can lead to severe inflammation and ulceration.

Side effects

The preparations of different strengths are all irritant and can produce soreness, swelling and inflammation. These side effects are more likely with stronger concentrations of podophyllin or if the application is not rinsed off the skin within a few hours. If the side effects are marked the patient may benefit from a small number of applications of a moderate potency topical steroid. This will help to minimize the symptoms of inflammation and may reduce the risk of extensive spread of warts into damaged skin (sometimes described as Köbnerization or Koebnerization), but should not be continued for any longer than absolutely necessary as it may encourage wart growth.

As podophyllin contains an anti-mitotic agent, there are theoretical risks of systemic effects if it is absorbed. This is more likely if a large area is treated with a strong solution or if it is applied to broken skin. Systemic toxicity has been reported with fatal outcome.[1] Its use is contraindicated in pregnancy as lower absorbed doses may have an effect on the fetus.

Expectations of treatment

The reported clearance rates for podophyllin treatment are rather variable and range between 20 and 80%. Recent studies have suggested that, after 4 or 5 weeks of weekly treatment, approximately 60% of females and nearly 80% of males were clear of warts.[2,3] Recurrence is not unusual and is of the order of 20–30% over the year after treatment.

Comparative studies of weekly clinic-applied podophyllin versus self-applied podophyllotoxin have given clearance rates and side-effect profiles in favour of podophyllotoxin (see the next section.)

Self-applied weak podophyllin solution (0.5 or 2%) has been compared to podophyllotoxin (0.5%) and found to lead to comparable rates of clearance of warts and side effects although no evaluation of recurrence was made.[4]

Podophyllotoxin

Method of treatment

Podophyllotoxin is available as 0.5% solution and 0.15% cream. Both the solution and the cream are for patient self-application. The solution can be used when the application sites can be easily seen, as in penile warts, whilst the cream may be easier to use for the vulval and peri-anal areas.

The podophyllotoxin preparation is applied twice a day to the affected skin for 3 consecutive days in a week. The 3-day treatment is repeated each week for 4–6 weeks. Unlike podophyllin, podophyllotoxin products do not have to be applied very accurately to only the warts. Some application to surrounding normal skin does not produce as much irritation as the unpurified podophyllin resin.

Side effects

The main side effects are due to irritation of the skin. The patient may report itching, tenderness, soreness or burning of the skin. Erythema, swelling and short-lived erosions may occur. These side effects are maximal on day 3 of each treatment cycle and often worst with the first cycle. If inflammation is severe with broken, superficially ulcerated skin, the treatment should be temporarily discontinued and then resumed with a reduction in the frequency of application.

The risk of teratogenicity should be assumed to apply to podophyllotoxin although there are no reports of fetal toxicity.

Expectations of treatment

A full course of treatment with podophyllotoxin cream is likely to result in the clearance of approximately 60–90% of warts in males and females.[2,5,6] The treatment is slightly less effective in the treatment of keratinized warts on areas of slightly thicker skin, so that in women and uncircumcised males the clearance rate may be nearer 50 or 60% after 4 weeks of treatment cycles. Warts in hair-bearing skin and in the urinary meatus may be less responsive to treatment.

The speed of clearance of warts with podophyllotoxin treatment is higher than with podophyllin[2] and the overall clearance rate is higher and the recurrence rate lower when the two therapies are compared directly.[2,3]

Individual warts that clear with podophyllotoxin treatment have a 10–40% chance of recurrence. The expected proportion of patients in whom clearance is sustained long-term after a single course of treatment is approximately 20%.

Use in children

Podophyllotoxin is not licensed in the UK for use in children. However, anecdotal accounts of its use have not suggested any different side effects and have supported its efficacy. It may be appropriate to use podophyllotoxin at a slightly lower frequency of application in young children. For instance some practitioners suggest application on just 2 days per week of each treatment cycle.

Fluorouracil

5-Fluorouracil (5-FU) is an anti-mitotic agent acting to halt or prevent cell division. It is used systemically in cancer chemotherapy, but as a topical or local application can act without systemic side effects.

A 5% cream formulation is available. This can be applied to warts, usually less frequently than daily. It is not recommended as a standard office treatment for warts, but it has been reported to be effective in a proportion of cases of cutaneous and mucosal ano-genital warts. It has been used for treating intra-urethral and meatal penile warts with reasonable success.[7]

An intra-lesional gel formulation is produced and is available in North America. It releases 5-FU more slowly from a bovine collagen gel containing adrenaline.

Method of treatment

The cream is applied to the affected area two or three times per week. The recommended treatment is for 6–10 weeks, but it may need to be used for 3 months. The intra-lesional gel is introduced by injection just at the base of the wart(s). The injection is painful.

Side effects

The cream can cause irritation. A vigorous response of irritation, soreness and occasionally erosion or ulceration may occur in some patients even when used only twice a week. Similar side effects are reported with the intra-lesional gel.

The agent is teratogenic when used in systemic therapy. This is probably not a major risk in topical treatment but it does mean that the treatment should not be used in pregnancy.

Expectations of treatment

A clearance rate of 40–70% is expected after 6 weeks of treatment. This is lower than the reported clearance with podophyllotoxin. However, the recurrence rates are similar, with approximately one-third of patients relapsing in the months after a course of treatment.

Cidofovir

Cidofovir acts by interfering with the production of new DNA in dividing cells or by a preferential effect on the production of new viral DNA within infected cells. The drug molecule becomes incorporated into DNA as it is forming and halts its formation. This then stops a cell dividing or, in the case of a virally infected cell in which only viral DNA is being produced, will stop the production of new viral DNA and, hence, interfere with new virus production. When used systemically, cidofovir has toxic side effects, but it is now being formulated as a topical therapy with more promising results for treatment of human papillomavirus (HPV) disease. At present, this treatment is only being used in a research setting.

Method of treatment
Cidofovir has been used experimentally as a 1% cream or gel, applied 5 days per week for up to 6 weeks.

Side effects
The treatment produces inflammation and discomfort and may lead to erosions and ulceration.

Expectations of treatment
A clearance rate of 70% has been achieved in patients with human immunodeficiency virus disease.[8] Clearance might be better in immunocompetent individuals, but so far no large studies have been performed.

Retinoids
Chemically related to vitamin A, the oral retinoids acitretin and 13-*cis*-retinoic acid have an anti-proliferative effect on the epidermis. They can act to reduce the size of warts, but do not necessarily clear the viral infection.

Method of treatment
The oral retinoids are given under specialist supervision. A dose of 0.5–1 mg/kg/day for up to 4 months is the usual regime.

Side effects
Retinoids can induce hepatitis, hyperlipidaemia and other symptoms of dry skin, hair loss and muscular aches. They are teratogenic and should only be taken by females who are also using adequate contraception.

Expectations of treatment
There are few reports of this treatment in genital warts, but in one recent study using isotretinoin at a dose of 1 mg/kg/day for 3 months clearance occurred in 18 out of 24 patients (33%).[9]

Destructive treatment

Trichloroacetic acid
This acts as a caustic, producing an effect of chemical cautery. It is applied as an 80–90% solution.

The treatment is not teratogenic and can be used or continued during pregnancy.

Method of treatment
The liquid is applied accurately to the warts. An orange stick, with or without a tight swab of cotton wool wrapped around the end produces an applicator that allows carefully controlled application. As long as the cotton wool tip is not too large and is wrapped firmly at the end, the risk of drips onto normal skin will be minimized. Application produces immediate damage to the living tissue, which turns whitish with a blue–green tinge. If spilt accidentally onto the skin immediate neutralization with an alkaline solution such as sodium bicarbonate will minimize unnecessary damage.

Trichloroacetic acid is applied weekly for the treatment of warts, although this can be slightly less frequent if the tissue response is vigorous. Three or four applications are often necessary in order to produce the clearance of warts.

Side effects
The application is painful, causing a burning, stinging feeling. The discomfort is often intense for 10–15 min after application, but can be painful for several hours. Many patients find the pain on application intolerable. Superficial erosions or ulcers may be left as the damaged skin separates. These will heal over a few days. Scarring is rare but may develop after deep ulceration or if there is secondary infection of the treated site.

Expectations of treatment
At the end of a treatment course, 70–80% of patients would expect to be clear of warts.[10] The reported recurrence rates vary between 30 and 60%.

Monochloroacetic acid

This is a very potent caustic agent. It is available as a moist crystalline compound and can be applied carefully in small quantities directly to individual warts. The application is painful. Over-treatment can result in deep ulceration. Treatment is usually repeated after full healing.

Cryotherapy

Cryotherapy is a method of destructive treatment. The use of liquid nitrogen as a spray, applied with a cotton wool bud or as a cooled probe, produces a means of freezing tissue. The frozen cells expand and lyse with subsequent necrosis and inflammation. Although this is a quick and easy method of damaging skin, it is difficult to control the depth of freezing precisely.

Method of treatment

Liquid nitrogen at a temperature of −196°C is the most commonly used method of freezing. The liquid can be used from an insulated vessel and applied by a dipped cotton wool bud directly onto the wart. Repeated transfer of the cotton wool bud from wart to liquid nitrogen is best avoided as the virus can be transferred into the stock of liquid nitrogen. An alternative method is to use a spray gun to apply the liquid onto the tissue. This avoids direct contact with the virus-infected skin and is somewhat quicker than the cotton wool bud method. The spray nozzle is available in a variety of sizes, thus allowing a smaller or larger area to be treated at a time. Finally, liquid nitrogen via the spray apparatus can be used to cool a solid probe, which can be applied directly to the skin. This enables warts in areas such as the vagina to be treated, when the spray technique would result in nitrogen cloud formation and obscured sight of the treated area. However, application of the probe to the skin, particularly if the skin or mucosa is slightly damp, can result in temporary sticking of the probe to the surface. As the treated area thaws out, the probe comes free.

Other methods of therapeutic freezing of the skin are carbon dioxide snow and dimethyl ether spray. Neither of these produces such a cold freeze as liquid nitrogen. They are therefore somewhat less destructive than liquid nitrogen, but also less effective.

In order to produce adequate freezing for destruction of tissue, the skin must be frozen and kept frozen for 15–20 s. Continuous freezing of 30 s or more is likely to result in ulceration or scarring and should thus be avoided. A greater tissue destructive effect is achieved if the tissue is frozen, thawed and frozen again.

Ideally, warts should be frozen at intervals of 1–3 weeks. A lower response rate results with longer intervals between freezing of the warts. Regular treatments may often need to be carried out for at least 3 months. This is of course a major commitment for both the patient and doctor or nurse.

Cryotherapy may be carried out without anaesthesia of the skin, but if the area to be frozen is extensive this may facilitate adequate tissue freezing.

Side effects
The procedure of freezing is painful. Initially there is a sensation of stinging cold, followed by a more intense pain that lasts approximately 1 min. Immediately after freezing the treated area will sting and become slightly pink and swollen. The first 30–60 min after freezing is quite painful and then the discomfort gradually settles over the rest of the day. The freezing is likely to produce some degree of tissue damage. This may cause the expected necrosis of the wart, but may also lead to superficial erosion or ulceration of the treated site. In some cases, a blister may form at the site of freezing.

The damage produced by the freezing may affect melanocytes causing depigmentation of dark skin.

Expectations of treatment
The clearance rates are reported to be 40–90%.[11,12] Approximately 70% clear at 3 months even after up to three freezes at weekly intervals. The recurrence rates may be

relatively high, with 30–60% of patients developing recurrent warts by 3 months after a course of treatment.

Photodynamic therapy

Photodynamic therapy involves the delivery of a substance to target tissue and the activation of that substance to a toxin by means of light. Photodynamic therapy is being developed for the treatment of genital warts, but is still at a research stage. The most commonly used phototoxic substance is protoporphyrin, part of the porphyrin metabolic cascade. It is usually delivered to the skin in the form of a precursor, amino-laevulinic acid (ALA), where normal cellular pathways then convert it into protoporphyrin. When the skin is then exposed to laser or visible light, this then 'activates' the metabolite of ALA into damaging the cells in which it is present.

Method of treatment

The ALA can be incorporated into a cream formulation that is applied to the skin for approximately 2 h, during which time it is taken up by abnormal or relatively rapidly dividing cells. The skin is then exposed to blue or laser light.

Side effects

The light exposure of the ALA-treated area can be a very painful experience and adequate pain control may be necessary.

Expectations of treatment

The treatment was well tolerated in a small study of 16 patients with genital warts and resulted in clearance in two-thirds of those receiving a single treatment.[13] The recurrence rate is unknown.

Surgery

Surgical removal of ano-genital warts depends on the site and size of the lesions. It may also be determined by patient acceptability and the success with other approaches. The idea is to remove the epidermis in which the papillomavirus is producing its effects. The virus does not infect the dermis so it is only necessary to remove infected epidermis. Damage to the dermo-epidermal junction will lead to scarring. The surgical approach does not necessarily remove the virus and does not treat subclinical papillomavirus infection.

Expectations of treatment

All visible disease can be treated using these methods, leading to a potential 100% clearance rate. Recurrences occur in approximately 10% within 3 months and in one-quarter of patients by 6 months.

Scissor snip

Method of treatment

This is a useful method of removal of protuberant warts. The warts and adjacent skin must first be anaesthetized before the wart is lifted away from the skin surface and snipped off with sharp scissors. Bleeding can be controlled with electrocautery.

Side effects

The procedure is likely to leave some scarring.

Curettage and cautery

Method of treatment

Once the skin affected with a wart is anaesthetized, the protuberant viral growth can be removed by curettage. The spoon-shaped curette is available as a disposable, sharp-edged instrument (Figure 4.1a) or as a relatively blunt-edged, sterilizable Volkmann's spoon (Figure 4.1b). The wart is scooped or scraped off the surface. The use of the blunter instrument depends upon the good plane of cleavage between the wart and normal skin.

Flatter or less exuberant warts can be treated surgically just by destructive burning of the abnormal skin. Again, adequate anaesthesia is required. A hot wire loop or diathermy with electrofulgation will singe and char the wart. The burnt eschar can be removed with a curette or scraped off with a scalpel blade.

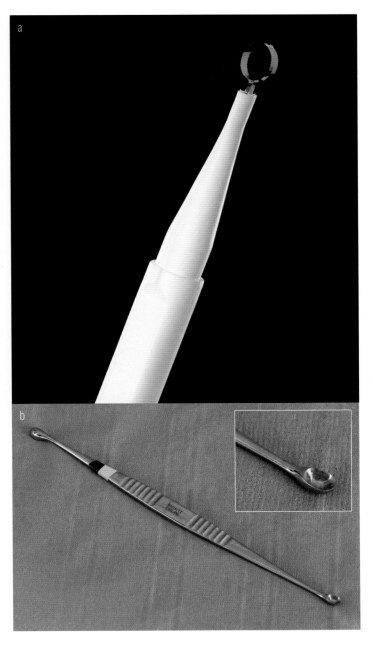

Figure 4.1
(a) Disposable
curette. (b)
Volkmann's spoon, a
sterilizable curette.

Side effects

There is a risk of pulling off adjacent, normal skin if the skin is fragile. The sharper, disposable loop curette allows a cleaner cut through at the base of the wart, although it may be easy to slice slightly deeper than intended. After the wart is removed, the base will bleed or ooze, necessitating cautery with electrodessication, hot wire cautery or chemical cautery.

Laser

Method of treatment

The carbon dioxide laser produces energy that causes a superficial destruction of the treated site. The laser application is painful and some form of anaesthesia is necessary. Genital warts can usually be treated in one session, but more extensive disease may need a total of two or three treatments.

Side effects

Ulceration resulting from the damage to superficial tissue may lead to secondary infection and occasionally cellulitis. Healing after laser treatment usually takes 2–3 weeks.

Immune stimulation

Boosting the immune system with the aim of stimulating rejection of the virus has been proposed as a potential treatment for genital warts. The most effective of these is topically applied imiquimod. At present, systemic treatments for modifying the immune response have not been proven to be very effective as single treatments.

Imiquimod

Imiquimod is an imidazoquinoline and acts by inducing inflammatory cytokines, particularly interferon (IFN), tumour necrosis factor-α and certain interleukins. It is licensed for the treatment of genital warts, but has also been shown to have a useful effect in superficial basal cell carcinoma and actinic keratoses. It is available in a cream formulation in small sachets that are for single use. The cream from a sachet will cover approximately 10 cm².

Method of treatment
The 5% cream is applied three times per week for up to 16 weeks. It is applied before sleep and followed by gentle washing on rising. Patients can apply the cream themselves.

Side effects
Most patients experience some side effects of treatment. Approximately two-thirds will find that their skin is inflamed, itchy or burning. This is tolerable for most people, but up to 10% may find the discomfort unacceptable. In this situation the cream can be discontinued for one or two applications and therapy restarted.

The drug has not been found to be harmful to the fetus in animals, but the cream is not licensed for use during pregnancy.

Expectations of treatment
At the end of a course of treatment, 40–60% of patients will be clear of warts, with over 70% showing at least partial clearance.[14,15,16] The clearance rates for treated women are higher (70-75%) than for men (35-60%)[17,18,19]. Recurrences seem to be slightly less likely than with other topical treatments. Approximately 10-20% of cleared patients suffer a recurrence of the warts by 3 to 6 months[14,19].

Interferons
IFNs are naturally produced chemicals that are released by virus-infected cells and help the body in containing and clearing a virus infection. IFN-α, IFN-β and IFN-γ have been produced for therapeutic use. All can be administered systemically as intravenous or intramuscular injections.

Intra-lesional injection can also be a useful method of delivery directly into warts. This permits a lower dose to be used with a subsequent reduction in systemic side effects. IFN-α has also been tried experimentally as a cream.

Method of treatment

IFN-α or IFN-γ at a dose of 3×10^6 U is given intra-lesionally once a week for 6 weeks or three times per week for 3 weeks.

Side effects

Generalized malaise, muscular aches and pains and headaches are common symptoms after systemic IFN administration. The side effects may last for 48 h after treatment. Similar feelings can be experienced after intra-lesional injection, but these are usually milder.

Expectations of treatment

Some early studies gave promising results for the use of IFNs, but as more randomized and placebo-controlled studies were reported the success rate was less impressive. Complete clearance after intra-lesional IFN alone occurs in approximately 15% of patients, which is a similar rate to that expected with placebo.[20] The reported recurrence rate is between 0 and 45%.

IFNs have been used in combination with other therapies and may offer some extra benefit.

The addition of IFN did not improve the overall outcome when used together with a carbon dioxide laser or cryotherapy.[21] However, the combination of IFN with topical fluorouracil or oral retinoid minimally improved the response rate.[9,22]

Cimetidine

This well-known histamine (H_2-receptor) blocker, which is used for the treatment of gastric irritation and ulceration, has some effects on T cell function. For this reason it has been tested as a treatment for warts.

Method of treatment

Cimetidine tablets are taken daily for approximately 3 months. The dosage is of the order of 30–40 mg/kg/day, that is approximately 400 mg three times per day in an adult.

Side effects
The side effects are minimal, but at this high dose some may experience malaise, dizziness or headaches.

Expectations of treatment
Reports of the efficacy of cimetidine in stimulating the clearance of skin or genital warts[23,24] were not borne out when the drug was used in placebo-controlled trials.[25,26] Its role in therapy is currently not clear.

Vaccination

Prophylactic and therapeutic vaccination for HPV infection is currently under development. A trial of vaccine against HPV 16, the type of HPV that is associated with cervical cancer, has shown promise[27] with apparent good protection against infection, at least in the short term. It may be that this success will trigger the development of a similar prophylactic approach against other HPV types including the causes of genital warts.

Treatment of established disease with a therapeutic vaccine has also been attempted.[28] A vaccine consisting of two proteins from HPV type 6 was used in 25 patients with genital warts. The warts cleared in five (20%) patients within 8 weeks and a further eight patients were cleared after additional conventional treatment. However, this result is not greatly different to an expected placebo response and further immunological advances will be needed before this can become an effective treatment.

Alternative therapies for the treatment of genital warts

Many possibilities exist for alternative therapy for the treatment of warts. Most prominent are treatments such as a homeopathic approach to boosting immune responses or herbalism using certain plants with potential effects on the skin. Numerous other suggestions can be found via the Internet. As yet, convincing evidence for their efficacy is lacking. Placebo-controlled trials of homeopathic treatment of cutaneous warts have not given encouraging results.[29,30]

Approaches to treating a patient with genital warts

When a person develops genital tumours that could be warts, it is sensible for the diagnosis to be made by a doctor or nurse. In addition, the patient should be screened for other sexually transmitted diseases. This will probably best be done at a sexual health or genitourinary medicine clinic. Once a diagnosis of genital warts is made, the choice of treatment will depend on many factors, depending on the extent and site of the disease, the patient's general health and also patient preference (Tables 4.2–4.4). Treatment will usually be started with topical

Table 4.2
Treatments used
commonly or rarely
for genital warts:
dose and method
of treatment.
(Treatments in
routine use are
indicated in Table
4.1).

Treatment	Formulation	Method of use
Local application		
Podophyllin	15–25% in tincture of benzoin compound	Weekly for 4–5 weeks: wash off after 4–8 hours
Podophyllotoxin	0.5% alcoholic solution or 0.15% cream	Twice a day for 3 consecutive days in a week, repeated for 4–6 weeks
5-FU	5% cream	Two or three times per week for 6–10 weeks
Trichloroacetic acid	80–90% solution	Weekly for 3–4 weeks
Monochloroacetic acid	Crystalline solution	Single application
Imiquimod	5% cream	Three times per week for up to 16 weeks
Local injection		
IFN	3×10^6 U IFN-α or IFN-γ	Intra-lesional injection once a week for 6 weeks or three times per week for 3 weeks
Local surgery		
Cryotherapy	–	15–20-s freeze, repeated every 1–3 weeks for 3 months
Curettage and scissor snip	–	Single surgical treatment that can be repeated
Laser	Carbon dioxide laser	Single treatment that can be repeated
Systemic		
Cimetidine	200 mg tablets	300–400 mg/day for 12 weeks
Retinoids	Isotretinoin and acitretin	0.5–1 mg/kg/day for 3–4 months

Treatment	Formulation	Side effects
Local application		
Podophyllin	15–25% in tincture of benzoin compound	Irritation, soreness, erosion and ulceration, systemic toxicity possible. Not for use in pregnancy
Podophyllotoxin	0.5% alcoholic solution or 0.15% cream	Irritation, soreness, erosion and ulceration and not licensed for use in pregnancy
5-FU	5% cream	Irritation, soreness, erosion and ulceration
Trichloroacetic acid	80–90% solution	Pain on application, irritation, soreness, erosion and ulceration
Monochloroacetic acid	Crystalline solution	Pain on application, irritation, soreness, erosion and ulceration
Imiquimod	5% cream	Irritation, soreness, erosion and ulceration
Local injection		
IFN	3×10^6 U IFN-α or IFN-γ	–
Local surgery		
Cryotherapy	–	Pain at time of use and for some while after, soreness, blistering, erosion and uleration
Curettage and scissor snip	–	–
Laser	Carbon dioxide laser	Pain, erosion and ulceration
Systemic		
Cimetidine	200 mg tablets	–
Retinoids	Isotretinoin and acitretin	Teratogenicity, hyperlipidaemia, hepatitis, and dry skin

Table 4.3
Treatments used commonly or rarely for genital warts: side effects. (Treatments in routine use are indicated in Table 4.1).

therapy, which is usually patient administered as long as the patient is able and compliant. A review for ensuring that there has been a response or for considering further treatment in the absence of a response is essential (Table 4.5). In addition, the patient should receive some information informing them about the potential infectious nature of warts.

Guidelines for treating patients with genital warts have been produced both in Europe and North America.[31,32] Although

Table 4.4
Treatments used
commonly or
rarely for genital
warts: clearance
and recurrence
rates. (Treatments
in routine use are
indicated in Table
4.1)

Treatment	Formulation	Clearance	Recurrence
Local application			
Imiquimod	5% cream	40–60%	10-20%
Podophyllin	15–25% in tincture of benzoin compound	60–80%	20–30% over the first year after treatment
Podophyllotoxin	0.5% alcoholic solution or 0.15% cream	60–90%	10–40%
5-FU	5% cream	40–70%	30% in the first year after treatment
Trichloroacetic acid	80–90% solution	70–80%	30–60%
Monochloroacetic acid	Crystalline solution	Not available	Not available
Local injection			
IFN	3×10^6 U IFN-α or IFN-γ	15%	0–45%
Local surgery			
Cryotherapy	–	70%	30–60% after 3 months
Curettage and scissor snip	–	–	10% at 3 months & 25% at 6 months
Laser	Carbon dioxide laser	Not available	Not available
Systemic			
Cimetidine	200 mg tablets	0–30%	Not available
Retinoids	Isotretinoin and acitretin	33%	Not available

there are slight differences in advice given, due to regional practices and therapy availability, both have the same messages with regard to the types of treatment that can be given.

References

1. Miller RA. Podophyllin. *Int J Dermatol* 1985; **24**: 491–8.
2. Kinghorn GR, McMillan A, Mulcahy F, Drake S, Lacey C, Bingham JS. An open, comparative study of the efficacy of 0.5% podophyllotoxin lotion and 25% podophyllin solution in the treatment of condylomata acuminata in males and females.

Application	Treatment
Patient-applied treatments	Podophyllotoxin solution or cream
	Weak podophyllotoxin (0.5–2%)
	Imiquimod cream
	5-FU cream
Patient-ingested therapy	Cimetidine
	Retinoid (supervised by specialist)
Doctor/Nurse-applied treatments	Podophyllin solution (15–25%)
	Trichloroacetic acid solution
	Monochloroacetic acid
	Photodynamic therapy
	Cryotherapy
	Scissor snip
	Curettage
	Laser
Doctor/Nurse-injected therapy	5-FU gel (North America)
	IFN

Table 4.5
Treatments: who can do what?

Int J STD AIDS 1993; **4**: 194–9.

3. Hellberg D, Svarrer T, Nilsson S, Valentin J. Self-treatment of female external genital warts with 0.5% podophyllotoxin cream (Condyline) vs weekly applications of 20% podophyllin solution. *Int J STD AIDS* 1995; **6**: 257–61.

4. White DJ, Billingham C, Chapman S *et al*. Podophyllin 0.5% or 2% v podophyllotoxin 0.5% for the self treatment of penile warts: a double blind randomised study. *Genitourinary Med* 1997; **73**: 184–7.

5. Bonnez W, Elswick RK, Bailey-Farchione A *et al*. Efficacy and safety of 0.5% podofilox solution in the treatment and suppression of genital warts. *Am J Med* 1994; **96**: 420–5.

6. Syed TA, Lundin S, Ahmad SA. Topical 0.3% and 0.5% podophyllotoxin cream for self-treatment of condylomata acuminata in women. A placebo-controlled, double-blind study. *Dermatology* 1994; **189**: 142–5.

7. Wein AJ, Benson GS. Treatment of urethral condyloma acuminatum with 5-fluorouracil cream. *Urology* 1977; **9**: 413–15.

8. Orlando G, Fasolo MM, Beretta R, Merli S, Cargnel A. Combined surgery and cidofovir is an effective treatment for genital warts in HIV-infected patients. *AIDS* 2002; **16**: 447–50

9. Cardamakis EK, Kotoulas IG, Dimopoulos DP, Stathopoulos EN, Michopoulos JT, Tzingounis VA. Comparative study of systemic interferon alfa-2a with oral isotretinoin and oral isotretinoin alone in the treatment of recurrent condylomata acuminata. *Arch Gynecol Obstet* 1996; **258**: 35–41.

10. Godley MJ, Bradbeer CS, Gellan M, Thin RNT. Cryotherapy compared with trichloroacetic acid in treating genital warts. *Genitourinary Med* 1987; **63**: 390–2.

11. Ghosh AK. Cryosurgery of genital warts in cases in which podophyllin treatment failed or was contraindicated. *Br J Venereol Dis* 1977; **53**: 49–53.

12. Simmons PD, Langlet F, Thin RNT. Cryotherapy versus electrocautery in the treatment of genital warts. *Br J Venereol Dis* 1981; **57**: 273–4.

13. Fehr MK, Hornung R, Degen A *et al*. Photodynamic therapy of vulvar and vaginal condyloma and intraepithelial neoplasia using topically applied 5-aminolevulinic acid. *Lasers Surg Med* 2002; **30**: 273–9.

14. Beutner KR, Spruance SL, Houghham AJ *et al*. Treatment of genital warts with an immune-response modifier (imiquimod). *J Am Acad Dermatol* 1998; **38**: 230-9.

15. O'Mahony C, Law C, Gollinck HPM, Marini M. New patient-applied therapy for anogenital warts is rated favourably by patients. *Int J STD AIDS* 2001; **12**: 565-70

16. Moore RA, Edwards JE, Hopwood J, Hicks D. Imiquimod for the treatment of genital warts: a quantitative systematic review. *BioMed Central Infect Dis* 2001; **1**(3): (http://www.biomedcentral.com/1471-2334/1/3).

17. Saunder DN, Skinner RB, Fox TL, Owens ML. Topical imiquimod 5% cream as an effective treatment for external genital and perianal warts in different patient populations. *Sex Trans Dis* 2003; **30**: 124-8.

18. Edwards L, Ferenczy A, Eron L *et al*. Self-administered topical 5% imiquimod cream for external anogenital warts. *Arch Dermatol* 1998; **134**: 25-30.

19. Garland SM, Sellors JW, Wikstrom A *et al*. Imiquimod 5% cream is a safe and effective self-applied treatment for

anogenital warts – results of an open-label, multicentre phase IIIB trial. *Int J STD AIDS* 2001; **12**: 722-9.

20. Trizna Z, Evans T, Bruce S, Hatch K, Tyring SK. A randomised phase II study comparing four different interferon therapies in patients with recalcitrant condylomata acuminata. *Sex Trans Dis* 1998; **25**: 361–5.

21. Bonnez W, Oakes D, Bailey-Farchione A *et al*. A randomised, double-blind trial of parenteral low dose versus high dose interferon-beta in combination with cryotherapy for treatment of condyloma acuminata. *Antiviral Res* 1997; **35**: 41–52.

22. Klutke JJ, Bergman A. Interferon as an adjuvant treatment for genital condylomata acuminatum. *Int J Gynaecol Obstet* 1995; **49**: 171–4.

23. Franco I. Oral cimetidine for the management of genital and perigenital warts in children. *J Urol* 2000; **164**: 1074–5.

24. Gooptu C, Higgins CR, James MP. Treatment of viral warts with cimetidine: an open label study. *Clin Exp Dermatol* 2000; **25**: 183–5.

25. Yilmaz E, Alpsoy E, Basaran E. Cimetidine therapy for warts: a placebo-controlled, double-blind study. *J Am Acad Dermatol* 1996; **34**: 1005–7.

26. Rogers CJ, Gibney MD, Siegfried EC, Harrison BR, Glaser DA. Cimetidine therapy for recalcitrant warts in adults: is it any better than placebo. *J Am Acad Dermatol* 1999; **41**: 123–7.

27. Koutsky LA, Ault KA, Wheeler CM *et al*. A controlled trial of human papillomavirus type 16 vaccine. *New Engl J Med* 2002; **347**: 1645–51.

28. Lacey CJ, Thompson HS, Monteiro EF *et al*. Phase IIa safety and immunogenicity of a therapeutic vaccine, TA-GW, in persons with genital warts. *J Infect Dis* 1999; **179**: 612–18.

29. Kainz JT, Kozel G, Haidvogl M, Smolle J. Homeopathic versus placebo therapy of children with warts on the hands: a randomised, double-blind clinical trial. *Dermatology* 1996: **195**; 318-20.

30. Labreque M, Audet D, Latulippe LG, Drouin J. Homeopathic treatment of plantar warts. *CanadianMedAssocJ* 1992: **146**; 1749–53.

31. Beutner KR, Reitano MV, Richwald GA, Wiley DJ and the American Medical Association Expert Panel on External Genital Warts. External genital warts: report of the American

Medical Association consensus conference. *Clin Infect Dis* 1998; **27**: 796–806.

32. Von Krogh G, Lacey CJN, Gross G, Barasso R, Schneider A. European course in HPV associated pathology: guidelines for primary care physicians for the diagnosis and management of anogenital warts. *Sex Transm Infect* 2000; **76**: 162–8.

Chapter 5

Management issues

Chris Sonnex

Why should we treat genital warts?

Since warts may resolve without treatment a case could be made for a 'wait-and-see' approach to management. Indeed some patients (and doctors) opt for non-intervention. Unfortunately warts may enlarge and spread before activation of an effective cell-mediated immune response, leading to regret that action was not taken earlier.

Reducing infectivity is often forwarded as a reason for removing warts, but the evidence for this assertion is not strong. Human papillomavirus (HPV) will often remain in the epithelium subclinically after warts have cleared and, although one would suspect that warts would shed more virus than subclinical infection, evidence is currently lacking.

HPV replication and viral load do increase from latent to subclinical to clinical infection, although the presumption of increasing infectivity from latent to clinical infection remains unproven. One study has shown that overt warts are more easily transmissible earlier than later in their natural history. The long incubation period for HPV infection before warts appear suggests that many transmission events may occur prior to the initiation of treatment. If this were the case then the treatment of warts would have little impact on transmission to partners. This was partly supported by an audit study that showed that the treatment of male sexual partners made no significant difference to the failure rate of treatment in women with genital warts. Treatment may prevent the infection of new sexual partners, but this remains unproven.

As mentioned previously, HPV produces a broad spectrum of disease, much of it subclinical. The high prevalence of HPV infection in the population and the fact that genital warts represent only the tip of the infection iceberg raises the question of the purpose of wart treatment. Most treatments are not specifically anti-viral (although imiquimod does produce an anti-viral effect by the generation of cytokines within the epithelium) and eradication of HPV by current treatment options is not an achievable goal.

Taking all of the above points into consideration, we arrive at the answer to the question of why treat genital warts. Patients and their sexual partners want them treated. Warts are cosmetically disfiguring and can lead to psychological morbidity.

Treatment considerations

Treatment choice is affected by the following.

1. Which treatments are available to the practitioner (e.g. is there access to cryotherapy, diathermy, etc.?).
2. Patient needs (e.g. unable to attend for regular treatment, unable to self-apply medication and requests a quick response to treatment).
3. Wart types and sizes and the numbers and sites of lesions. Although there is widespread agreement among clinicians on this approach, there are no well-designed treatment trials comparing outcomes at different sites or in relation to wart morphology. Treatment decisions are therefore frequently made on 'considered opinion'.

Lesion type

Keratinized warts

These types of warts are usually best treated by cryotherapy or a surgical approach, such as diathermy or scissor excision.

The response to topical agents such as imiquimod, podophyllotoxin and trichloracetic acid may be unsatisfactory or

Keypoints

* HPV produces a broad spectrum of disease
* Genital warts represent only the tip of the infection iceberg
* Most treatments are not specifically anti-viral (although imiquimod produces an anti-viral effect by the generation of cytokines within the epithelium)

slow, but self-applied treatments are certainly worth considering if lesions are multiple.

Imiquimod may prove an important first line treatment for genital warts if the early studies suggesting a lower recurrence rate are confirmed.[1]

Non-keratinized warts

These usually respond well to imiquimod and podophyllotoxin and should be considered as first-line treatments for easily accessible sites. Cryotherapy or trichloracetic acid (small lesions) may be used in cases where practitioner-delivered treatment is considered necessary (e.g. non-accessible sites or patient choice). Many genitourinary (GU) medicine clinicians use a combination treatment of cryotherapy plus podophyllin, although no studies have formally examined this approach.

Lesion number

Multiple warts are usually best approached by a topical self-applied treatment such as imiquimod or podophyllotoxin.

Imiquimod should be considered for the treatment of large areas as podophyllotoxin may cause quite marked soreness, although this has also been reported with imiquimod.

Cryotherapy can be used, but is time-consuming if large areas require treatment and may produce intolerable discomfort both during the procedure and following the treatment. The application of a topical anaesthetic (e.g. lignocaine gel or lignocaine–prilocaine (EMLA) cream) 20–30 minutes prior to cryotherapy helps to make the procedure more tolerable.

Multiple, large warts are often best suited to surgery. Scissor excision in combination with electrosurgery or laser ablation performed under general anaesthesia is probably ideal. An alternative approach is to remove lesions 'area by area' under local anaesthesia. The application of topical anaesthesia prior to injections of local anaesthetic allows the procedure to be performed as comfortably as possible and the warts can be cleared over a period of a few sessions (depending upon the area affected).

Small numbers of warts are best treated by cryotherapy, scissor excision or electrosurgery.

Lesion size

Large warts are usually best treated by surgical methods, in particular scissor excision. Pedunculated lesions are easily treated by this method with only minimal subsequent bleeding.

Small warts may be treated by any method although the site and number of lesions should be taken into consideration.

Lesion site
Penis and vulva
Treatment choice will be determined by the size, number and type of warts, as discussed above.

Urethral meatus
Imiquimod, podophyllotoxin, cryotherapy or electrosurgery may be used if the warts can be fully visualized. Meatoscopy is a useful method of assessing the extent of lesions. Electrosurgery and laser ablation may be performed under local anaesthetic through an auroscope using a metal rather than plastic 'earpiece'. Referral to a urology department is recommended if the warts extend into the urethra beyond view.

Vagina
Adequate visualisation of lesions can prove difficult without the use of a colposcope. For this reason, referral onto a GU medicine clinician is recommended. If treatment is to be provided in primary care, consider cryotherapy or trichloracetic acid (with care!). A practitioner may apply podophyllin alone, although it is currently recommended that no more than a total area of 2 cm^2 be treated at each session.

Keypoints

* Multiple warts are usually best approached by a topical self-applied treatment

* Cryotherapy can be used to treat multiple warts, but is time-consuming if large areas require treatment and may produce intolerable discomfort

* Multiple, large warts are usually best treated with surgery

Cervix

Cervical warts are found in approximately 6–8% of women with external genital warts. Colposcopic examination and biopsy should be performed before starting treatment since the presence of cervical intra-epithelial neoplasia (CIN) II/III in addition to condylomata warrants treatment by large loop excision of the transformation zone. Patients with histological evidence of HPV/CIN I may be treated by cryotherapy or trichloracetic acid. Some specialist units (i.e. GU medicine and gynaecology) remove cervical warts by laser ablation or loop excision.

Peri-anal

Imiquimod, podophyllotoxin cream or cryotherapy are appropriate first-line treatments. Electrosurgery, scissor excision or laser ablation are useful if the lesions are not too numerous, although the injection of local anaesthetic can prove most uncomfortable even after the application of EMLA cream.

Many clinicians would advise proctoscopy for patients with peri-anal warts in order to assess for anal canal lesions, although this is by no means routine practice.

Proctoscopy may be performed after the peri-anal warts have cleared and is particularly important if there is a history of anal bleeding.

Immunosuppressed patients with anal warts should be carefully checked for the presence of anal intra-epithelial neoplasia. Human immunodeficiency virus (HIV)-positive 'men who have sex with men' are at particular risk.

Intra-anal

Intra-anal warts often respond slowly to treatment, due in part to difficult access and subsequent failure to treat the total wart mass. The anal canal is optimally visualized by colposcopic examination via a proctoscope. Cryotherapy and trichloracetic acid are both appropriate first-line treatments. Electrosurgery and laser ablation are a little more difficult to use at this site as bleeding post-injection of local anaesthetic can obscure the view.

General issues regarding treatment

Try to use a treatment that is convenient for the patient and likely to clear the warts quickly. A few warts may be better approached by removal under local anaesthetic rather than have the patient self-apply medication or attend a clinic on two or more occasions for cryotherapy.

If the warts are numerous and non-keratinized, consider a self-applied treatment. Most patients prefer this to attending a clinic on a weekly basis for trichloracetic acid application or cryotherapy.

Patients should be provided with information about the condition, both verbally and supported by an information sheet or booklet.

Other management issues

Screening for other genital infections

Patients with genital warts should routinely undergo screening for other sexually transmitted infections. A retrospective study in the UK reported that 32% of men and 61% of women with genital warts had a coincident genital infection and in 29% of men and 28% of women this was a sexually transmitted infection.

Psychological issues

For some patients the psychological impact of having genital warts is the worst aspect of the disease. One study found that 52% of men and 61% of women were 'quite concerned' or 'very concerned' about having warts. Other studies have documented frequent reports of anxiety, depression, isolation, stigmatization, alienation, negative self-image, shame and sexual impairment. Concern that genital warts may become cancerous has been reported in 28% of patients and should be addressed at an early stage in treatment. The provision

Keypoints

❋ Most patients prefer a self-applied treatment

❋ Patients with genital warts should be screened for other sexually transmitted infections – a study revealed that 29% of men and 28% of women had a coincident infection

of clear information and an opportunity to talk at the time of diagnosis may help ease anxiety. Patients have expressed greater satisfaction with physician encounters in which they have been encouraged to talk about relevant psychosocial issues.

Cervical screening

Women with genital warts have been shown to have a higher risk of cervical infection with HPV types 16 and 18. One study comparing a normal control group of women with patients with warts or dyskaryosis on cervical cytology found a higher rate of high grade CIN in women with warts.[2] However, multivariate analysis showed that CIN II/III was significantly associated with HPV 16/18 rather than the presence of warts. The study also demonstrated that cervical cytology was an effective option for the detection of CIN II/III in women with genital warts. These findings can therefore be interpreted as being in support of the current UK recommendation that women with genital warts do not require more frequent cervical screening than women without warts.

Treatment of special groups

Pregnancy

Genital warts often enlarge and multiply during pregnancy. Treatment therefore aims to reduce neonatal exposure to virus and minimise patient discomfort, which can be appreciable with large lesions. Potential problems for children include the development of laryngeal papillomatosis and ano-genital warts. The risk of acquiring laryngeal papillomatosis has been estimated to be between one in 400 and less than one in 1000. However, there is no formal evidence that treating genital warts in the mother reduces this risk. Caesarean section may be indicated in women with large cervical or vaginal warts. Podophyllotoxin and podophyllin are contraindicated in pregnancy because of possible teratogenicity. In the case of imiquimod, animal teratology (rat and rabbit) and reproductive studies (rat), no teratogenic nor embryofoetotoxic effects have been observed. Data on a limited number of pregnancies are available but no general conclusion can currently be drawn from these. It is therefore recommended that caution should be exercised when prescribing imiquimod in pregnancy.

Response to treatment during pregnancy is often slow, particularly in the third trimester. Since genital warts often clear spontaneously post-partum, a wait-and-see policy may be used, bearing in mind that lesions may enlarge and spread. A reasonable approach would be to leave small lesions if the patient is not too concerned by their presence. Larger warts, particularly if located at the introitus or at the site of potential episiotomy, may be treated. Cryotherapy, trichloracetic acid for small lesions and scissor excision of large lesions are the most appropriate treatment options.

Immunosuppression

Immunosuppression can occur as a congenital disorder or may be acquired in life either spontaneously due to disease or iatrogenically. Individuals receiving long-term immunosuppressive therapy and those with HIV infection or other cell-mediated immune deficiencies are prone to develop multiple and intractable warts. Although standard regimes may be tried, response can be slow and relapse common. A surgical approach or a combination of cryotherapy and surgery is often required with close follow-up so that new lesions can be treated at an early stage. Imiquimod is one of the treatment modalities for genital warts that has been formally examined in HIV-infected patients and a >50% reduction in wart area was observed in 38% of imiquimod-treated patients compared to 14% of vehicle-treated patients ($p = 0.013$). Imiquimod may also have a useful role in post-organ transplant patients although discussion with the 'transplant team' is recommended prior to starting treatment. Organ transplantation with lungs, hearts or kidneys requires high, prolonged immunosuppression and the patients are at high risk of developing troublesome

Keypoints

✳ A surgical approach or a combination of cryotherapy and surgery is often required for individuals receiving long-term immunosuppressive therapy, those with HIV infection or other cell-mediated immune deficiencies

✳ Imiquimod is one of the treatment modalities for genital warts that has been examined in HIV-infected patients giving a >50% reduction in wart area in 38% of patients

warts. Liver transplant recipients often need only very low doses of immunosuppressive therapy within a year or two of transplantation and this group appears to have less trouble with post-transplant warts.

Lack or reduced levels of immunoglobulins alone with normal cell-mediated immunity, as in hypogammaglobulinaemia or myeloma, does not cause an increased susceptibility to warts or reduced clearance of the infection.

Children

Although ano-genital warts have been well documented in children there are no reliable data on their prevalence. The possibility of sexual abuse must be considered in all children with genital warts. However, other physical signs, behavioural problems, psychosocial and social conditions must be assessed and taken into consideration. For this reason, it is best that a specialist multidisciplinary team undertakes the evaluation of children with genital warts. Auto-inoculation of a child from hand warts or transfer from parental hand lesions during close family contact (e.g. bathing, toileting, etc.) has been suggested by reported cases of hand wart HPV types 2 and 3 in some children with genital warts. Peri-natal transmission has been considered a theoretical possibility, in much the same way as laryngeal papillomas caused by HPV type 11 are transmitted during passage through the mother's infected birth canal. Owing to the poor correlation between HPV type and wart morphology, clinical examination should not be relied upon for predicting HPV type. The role of HPV testing in determining HPV type in children with ano-genital warts is uncertain. From the discussion above, this would seem to be limited.

No study data are available for guiding the treatment of children with ano-genital warts. An initial period of observation is recommended, as a proportion of cases will resolve spontaneously.

If warts are persistent, treatment may be indicated. Treatments such as imiquimod and podophyllotoxin are

Keypoints

✻ In all children with genital warts, the possibility of sexual abuse should be evaluated by a specialist multidisciplinary team

not licensed for use in children. However, there are several anecdotal reports that they are effective and safe when used in youngsters. A frequency of application less than that recommended for adults has been used and will be less likely to produce irritation. Surgery, often under general anaesthetic for younger children, can be considered. Cryotherapy is often not tolerated by children, even after the application of an anaesthetising cream.

The elderly

Genital warts and indeed all warts are much rarer in older life than` in childhood and young adults. When occurring in the elderly, the warts can be slow to clear, either spontaneously or with treatment. Surgical removal may therefore be worth considering at an earlier stage.

Key points

1. Consider the wart type, site and number of lesions and the needs of the patient when deciding which treatment to use.
2. Many patients prefer self-treatment, which may be with imiquimod or podophyllotoxin.
3. Cryotherapy, electrocautery and surgical excision are excellent treatments for most warts.
4. Following wart clearance, recurrence is common with rates of between 25 and 67% within 3 months.
5. Individuals with HIV infection and other cell-mediated immune deficiencies are prone to develop multiple and intractable warts.
6. The possibility of sexual abuse must be considered in all children with genital warts. However, other physical signs, behavioural problems and psychosocial and social conditions must be assessed and taken into consideration.

References

1. Beutner KR, Tyring SK, Trofatter K *et al.* Imiquimod, a patient-applied immune-response modifier for treatment of external genital warts. *Antimicrobiol Agents Chemother* 1998; **42**: 789–94.
2. Lacey CJN, Monteiro EF, MacDermott RIJ, Gibson P. High grade CIN: associations and screening strategies. *Genitourinary Med* 1996; **72**: 304.

Recommended reading

Beutner KR, Reitano MV, Richwald GA, Wiley DJ and the American Medical Association Expert Panel on External Genital Warts. External genital warts: report of the American Medical Association Consensus Conference. *Clin Infect Dis* 1998; **27**: 796–806.

Mortality and Morbidity Weekly Reports. MMWR Recommendations and Reports. 1998; **47**: 1–118 (www.cdc.gov/ncidod/guidelines).

UK national guidelines on sexually transmitted infections and closely related conditions: anogenital warts. Clinical Effectiveness Group (Association of Genitourinary Medicine and the Medical Society for the Study of Venereal Diseases). *Sex Transm Infect* 1999; **75**(Suppl 1): S71–5 (updated in 2002: available at www.mssvd.org .uk).

Von Krogh G, Lacey CJN, Gross G, Barasso R, Schneider A. European course in HPV associated pathology: guidelines for primary care physicians for the diagnosis and management of anogenital warts. *Sex Transm Infect* 2000; **76**: 162–8.

Chapter 6
Case studies

Chris Sonnex and Jane Sterling

Question
This 22-year-old woman presented with localized vulval irritation and was concerned that the skin felt 'lumpy'. The small warts in Figure 6.1 were seen. How would you treat them?

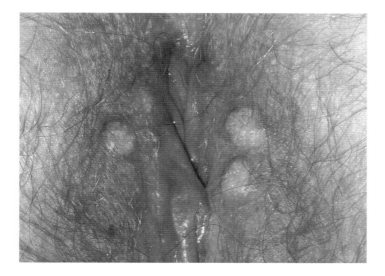

Figure 6.1
Vulval warts.

Answer
Cryotherapy or excision/electrocautery would be appropriate for such a small number of tiny warts. Self-applied treatments (such as imiquimod and podophyllotoxin) could be used if ablative methods were unavailable.

Question

This 31-year-old woman presented with a small, mildly itchy vulval lump (see Figure 6.2). How would you manage this case?

Figure 6.2
VIN.

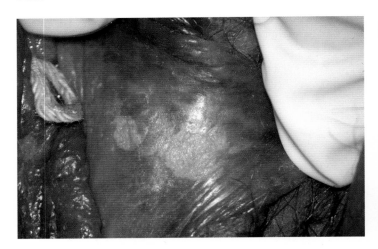

Answer

This is not a typical genital wart. The lesion is almost flat and is slightly pigmented. The appearances are consistent with a diagnosis of vulval intra-epithelial neoplasia (VIN) and, therefore, a biopsy should be performed before treating. If VIN is confirmed, local excision would be the most appropriate treatment. The message here is to consider biopsy (possibly via a clinician with an interest in vulval disease) if there is any doubt about the diagnosis. This is particularly important for flat or papular genital lesions.

Question

This 24-year-old man had noticed fresh blood on his underpants and occasional 'pink urine'. Neither the patient nor the general practitioner he initially consulted and who referred him on to a urology department with a view to performing cystoscopy had seen these intra-meatal warts. Intra-meatal warts may only be seen by everting the intra-epithelial epithelium, which is achieved by pressing firmly down with the thumbs on either side of the meatus (see Figure 6.3). How would you treat this patient?

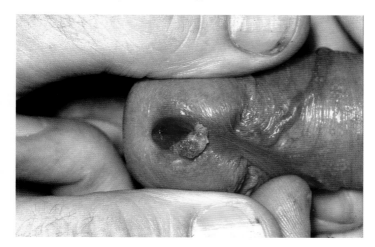

Figure 6.3
Intra-meatal warts.

Answer

Ablation by cryotherapy or electrocautery is an appropriate first-line treatment. Access to warts beyond the meatus may be achieved via the earpiece of an auroscope. Self-applied treatments (e.g. imiquimod or podophyllotoxin) could be used, although application may prove difficult if the meatus is small.

Question

This married man presented with anal irritation and received treatment for haemorrhoids. After 2 months without symptomatic improvement he was examined and peri-anal warts diagnosed (see Figure 6.4). What treatment would you recommend?

Figure 6.4
Peri-anal warts.

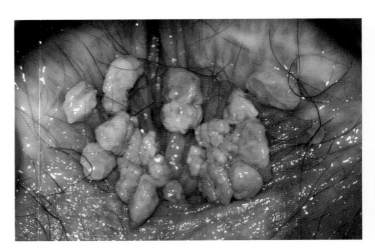

Answer

Self-applied imiquimod or podophyllotoxin would be appropriate. Both may cause soreness. The extent of the lesions makes cryotherapy a less attractive choice. Removal by scissor excision under local anaesthetic (or general anaesthetic following surgical referral) should also be considered.

Question

This 26-year-old married woman presented with post-coital bleeding (see Figure 6.5). How would you manage this case?

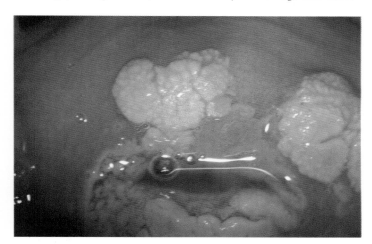

Figure 6.5
Cervical warts.

Answer

Refer for colposcopy. A full colposcopic examination is required as occasionally high-grade cervical intra-epithelial neoplasia may be present alongside cervical warts, in which case loop excision of the transformation zone would be the most appropriate treatment.

Question

A 30-year-old man presented with the small penile warts shown in Figure 6.6. What treatment would you recommend?

Figure 6.6
Penile warts.

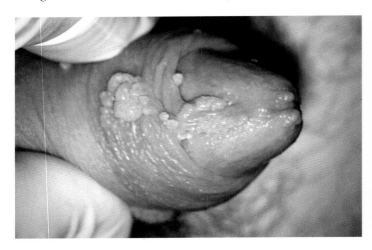

Answer

These are ideally suited to self-treatment with either imiquimod or podophyllotoxin. Both may cause soreness, in which case treatment should be deferred until the symptoms have settled.

Question

A middle-aged man presents with penile warts. He denies any extramarital sexual contact for at least 10 years and his wife does not have warts. Is it possible that he could have carried the virus for this length of time?

Answer

It is possible for the human papillomavirus to remain hidden in the skin for many years, even without the presence of visible warts. The exact length of time that the virus can remain in this latent state is not known. It would be sensible to check that there is no immunosuppression that could have triggered the appearance of the disease. In case the full sexual history has not been disclosed, it is advisable to check for other sexually transmitted infections.

Question

A five-year-old girl develops a few small warts over the peri-anal skin. They cause some irritation. Is this an indication of sexual abuse? How should the child/family be investigated? What treatment is best for the girl?

Answer

Warts in the ano-genital area are, by themselves, not proof of sexual abuse, but they can be an indicator of abuse. If there are other signs of possible abuse, such as bruising or fissuring in the genital area or abnormal behaviour of the child, then the possibility of abuse must be seriously entertained and appropriate steps taken to investigate this. Referral to and assessment by a paediatrician trained in this field is recommended. The treatment of ano-genital warts in a child may not be necessary as spontaneous regression may occur. Possible treatments to consider are topical imiquimod, podophyllotoxin or surgery (see page 87).

Question

A thirty-year-old man has had recurrent penile warts over the last 5 years. He and his partner wish to start a family. What treatment should or should not be used for the man at this time? Should you examine or investigate his partner?

Answer

Any of the treatments used for genital warts can be used. Podophyllotoxin and podophyllin should not be used in a woman planning pregnancy, but can be used in the man, provided of course that the treatment is washed off before intercourse. As genital warts in a woman can worsen during pregnancy, it may be of use to examine the partner and treat any warts before the pregnancy commences.

Chapter 7
Frequently asked questions

Chris Sonnex and Jane Sterling

Are genital warts always sexually transmitted?

The majority of genital warts are acquired as a result of sexual intercourse. Hand wart human papillomavirus (HPV) types have been reported to cause genital lesions in children, but this is uncommon in adults. Genital HPV types have been detected on the fingers of patients with genital warts, but this does not necessarily indicate transmission from the hands to genitals. Similarly, although HPV DNA has been found on underwear and examination gloves, there is no evidence to suggest that the virus can be transmitted from these contaminated objects.

How can I tell whom I caught them from?

This can sometimes prove difficult because of the potentially long incubation period between acquiring the infection and warts appearing. Although the average time is 3 months, much longer periods have been documented. If a partner has genital warts and there have been no other sexual contacts in the previous few months, the likelihood is that they have been caught from that sexual partner. The difficulty is when the current partner has no history of warts. It is recommended that partners should be examined as not infrequently small warts may found by the clinician, the patient being totally unaware of their presence. If warts are detected, it can still prove difficult to say who passed on the virus, unless perhaps there is a past history of genital warts in one or other of the partners. When no warts are found in the partner, the most diplomatic approach is to tell the patient that it is impossible to know when the infection was acquired. A patient presenting with first-episode genital warts and who denies any type of sexual contact within the previous several years is uncommon but familiar to most genitourinary medicine clinicians.

If I have sex when I have warts will I always pass on the virus?

In research over 30 years ago, Oriel[1] studied the partners of patients with genital warts over a period of months. Of just under 100 contacts examined, 64% developed warts after an interval of 3 weeks to 8 months (average 2.8 months). This was performed without the use of a colposcope, which may possibly have detected more cases.

There is some evidence to suggest that warts are most infectious shortly after their appearance.

Am I still infectious after the warts have disappeared?

When the visible 'bumps' of genital warts have disappeared naturally or after treatment, sometimes the DNA of the virus can still be found on the skin by sensitive detection methods (DNA hybridization techniques, e.g. the polymerase chain reaction). The same detection methods can sometimes also reveal the presence of the virus even before any disease develops. This means that there is a small chance of still being infectious even after the visible warts have gone.

How likely am I to pass on the virus if I have sex when I am just carrying the virus subclinically?

The infectivity of HPV is related to the viral copy number. The infectivity of subclinical infection is thought to be less than in overt disease as the viral load is low in latent infection and restricted to the epithelial basal layer. This is an assumption. However, the high prevalence of HPV infection in young sexually active adults without genital warts suggests that transmission does occur from subclinical infection.

Should I use condoms?

For patients with genital warts using condoms with regular sexual partners may reduce the development of new lesions, but this does not appear to affect treatment outcome. Although a number of studies have suggested that condom usage does not reduce the risk of HPV transmission to partners, one study has suggested a protective effect in men. A study from Australia looked at individuals without warts and found that, for both sexes, a failure to use condoms was independently associated with an increased risk of the acquisition of genital warts and that consistent condom use was associated with a decreased risk of acquiring genital warts.

Most patients prefer to use condoms whilst visible warts are present. The need for using condoms after wart clearance is uncertain. Some clinicians advise condom usage for 2–3 months after clearance, as warts are more likely to recur during this time. However, the use of condoms for preventing the transmission of subclinical infection has not been established and there is therefore no evidence to support the advice to use condoms once warts have gone. As the long-term sexual partners of individuals with warts are likely to have already been infected with HPV 6 or 11 there would appear to be little need for continuing to use condoms after warts have cleared.

Will the wart treatment alter condom efficiency?

The topical treatments for genital warts should not damage latex. However, it would be wise to allow podophyllotoxin lotion to dry and for podophyllotoxin cream and imiquimod cream to be absorbed into the skin before using a condom as this could spread the preparation to non-affected sites.

Do genital warts mean that I am likely to get cervical cancer?

Only some of the 100 or so different types of HPV have the potential for producing a risk of developing cancer in the genital area. These so-called 'high-risk' types are not the types that are responsible for causing genital warts. Current evidence suggests that women with genital warts are no more likely to develop cervical cancer than women without warts and therefore do not require more intensive cervical screening. One study reported an increased risk of cancer in the anal and genital areas, particularly vulval cancer, in women who had been hospitalized for wart treatment.

Can I or my partner catch cancer?

The high-risk HPV types associated with ano-genital cancer are sexually acquired and are usually carried subclinically in the epithelium, i.e. without having any signs of disease. The majority of these infections are transient and, of those infections that persist, the risk of developing cancer is very small. A number of factors influence the risk of developing cancer, such as smoking, genetics and the way your immune system copes with the virus.

Can I start a family while warts are present?

The presence of genital warts in either the man or the women will not alter fertility and will not increase the risk of having an abnormal baby. Some treatments used for genital warts should not be used during pregnancy, so if you are planning a pregnancy, you should tell the doctor who is treating you. Treatments to be avoided during pregnancy are podophyllotoxin, podophyllin and tablet treatments such as retinoids. Genital warts in a woman can often get bigger during pregnancy although they usually improve again after delivery. If warts are large or are affecting the cervix or vagina at the time of delivery, Caesarean section may be recommended because of the risk of bleeding if any tears occur during labour. There is a small chance of the wart infection from the mother being passed on to the baby at the time of delivery. This risk is thought to be between one in 400 and one in 1000 and does not warrant Caesarean section.

I or my partner have/have had genital warts. How often should I have a cervical smear?

You should have a cervical smear as recommended by national guidelines. This varies between countries but will usually be every 1–5 years. There is no need to have more frequent cervical smears if you have genital warts, nor is it recommended if you have been in contact with an infected partner. If any smear shows an abnormality, you will be asked to have another smear after 6 months or be referred for colposcopic examination of the cervix, depending upon the degree of abnormality detected.

I have/have had genital warts. Can I have oral sex?

If you have warts and your partner's mouth comes into direct contact with the warts, there is a chance that the warts could spread to your partner's lips or inside the mouth. It is therefore usually recommended to refrain from oral sex while warts are present. The risk of warts speading from one person to another in this way is probably the same as from person to person practising genital to genital sex without the use of a condom. It may be possible to avoid contact with warts during oral sex, if sufficient care is taken!

Can I do anything else to help myself?

Your body's immune system is best able to combat genital warts if you are generally well. If you are 'run down' and very tired or stressed, then your immune system may not be functioning maximally. Although there is no firm evidence that changes in diet or life style make any significant difference to the clearance of warts, it is a good idea to eat healthily and get enough sleep. People who smoke are more likely to have a small but definite increased risk of developing cervical cancer or vulval cancer if they are carrying a 'high-risk' type of HPV than people who do not smoke.

Reference

1. Oriel JD. Natural history of genital warts. *Br J Venereal Diseases* 1971; **47**: 1–13.

3